The Aromatherapy Handbook: Essential Oils Uses and Applications

by Marian Johnson

Disclaimer:

The information contained in this book is for general information purposes only. The statements contained herein have not been evaluated nor approved by the US Food and Drug Administration. This book is sold with the understanding the author and/or publisher is not giving medical advice, nor should the information contained in this book replace medical advice, nor is it intended to diagnose or treat any disease, illness or other medical condition. Always seek the advice of your physician or a qualified health provider prior to starting any new treatment or if you have any questions regarding a medical condition.

All recommendations contained herein are believed to be effective, but the effectiveness has not been evaluated and no guarantees are made or implied nor is any liability taken. Use essential oils at your own risk and never use them to treat ailments against the advice of a qualified medical professional.

While we endeavor to keep the information up to date and correct, we make no representations or warranties of any kind, express or implied, about the completeness, accuracy, reliability, suitability or availability with respect to the book or the information, products, services, or related graphics contained book for any purpose. Any reliance you place on such information is therefore strictly at your own risk.

The information contained herein should not be considered to be complete. There may be safety concerns not mentioned in the book that you need to be aware of. Consult with your doctor or physician prior to using any essential oil or aromatherapy treatment.

Dedication:

It was a long time coming, but I finally finished the book I've been thinking of writing for years. I couldn't have done it without the support and help of my friends and family, or as I like to call them, my guinea pigs. Thanks for letting me test new concoctions out on you guys.

Contents

Aromatherapy and How It Can Help You

Aromatherapy involves the use of essential oils and other plant-based compounds to help rebalance the human mind, body and soul. It's an all-natural approach to treatment, as opposed to the chemical compounds and invasive procedures relied upon in Western medicine. While there are detractors who would have you believe aromatherapists are selling nothing more than snake oil, there is an ever-growing group of believers who have used essential oils and have seen and felt exactly how powerful they are.

Aromatherapy is used to promote both physical and emotional health and well-being. While it would be a lie to claim essential oils can be used to cure all your ills, it isn't too much of a stretch to state they can be used in conjunction with—and at times, instead of—Western medicine to take care of a number of emotional and physical issues.

Essential oils, also known as volatile or ethereal oils, are oils derived from organic plant matter. They are the concentrated aromatic essence of the plant they've been extracted from. These oils give a plant its distinctive smell. In addition to scent, essential oils contain a number of naturally-occurring compounds that are known to be beneficial to the human body. They're packed with nutrients, vitamins, minerals and all sorts of other helpful chemicals that aid the body in a number of ways. Best of all, they're entirely natural and the body treats them as such.

To understand the intent behind aromatherapy, all you have to do is break the word apart. "Aroma" means fragrance and "therapy" means treatment. Aromatherapy at its core seeks to treat a variety of conditions through use of natural plant oils that rebalance the body and leave you feeling healthy and refreshed.

Inhalation of the fragrances of essential oils is one of the main applications of aromatherapy. In addition to inhalation, oils can be applied topically and some oils can even be ingested in small amounts. Depending on the method of application, essential oils can interact with your body in the following ways:

- **They can rebalance and adjust your internal chemistry by adding beneficial chemicals and removing toxins.**
- **They travel through the body and aid with the internal functions.**
- **They act directly on the area to which they are applied.**
- **They improve your mental health and state of mind.**

The true power behind aromatherapy lies in the fact that it acts on all of these aspects simultaneously. You get better, feel better and improve your body's overall health in the process.

Western medicine, on the other hand, consists of harsh medications and invasive procedures to treat illnesses and ailments. While these treatments may be necessary to treat larger health issues that can't be alleviated through use of aromatherapy, minor health issues are likely better off being treated naturally. It isn't uncommon for an almost-healthy person to start taking a prescription medication and to have a reaction to it. The doctor does what he's been trained to do and prescribes more medicine to take care of the side effects of the first medicine. When more problems arise, more medications are prescribed. Soon, the person is so chemically unbalanced that bigger problems start to p[op up—problems that may not have shown their ugly face had the patient not pounded his or her body with a constant barrage of synthetic medications.

I saw this take place first-hand with my father. He injured his back at work and was prescribed a relatively light prescription of codeine to ease his pain. The codeine caused nausea and his blood pressure spiked, so instead of taking my dad off the codeine, the doctor prescribed more medications to take care of the new problems. Insomnia set in and sleeping pills were prescribed, along with valium to help him relax. Before long, the man who I'd never seen take a pill in his life was popping more pills than Charlie Sheen on a bender. It was tough on his body and even tougher on his family to watch him go through it. Whenever we tried to talk to him about it, all he did was claim it was fine because the doctor prescribed it. He popped pills until his dying day, when his body collapsed under the heavy burden he'd been placing on it for decades.

This sort of overmedicating takes place across the globe. You'd be hard-pressed to find a person who doesn't at least know someone who's been medicated to the point of incoherence by doctors practicing modern medicine.

A number of problems that doctors typically prescribe medication for can often be treated through aromatherapy. While I'd never suggest stopping use of modern medicine altogether to treat serious illnesses and ailments, I do suggest discussing natural treatments with both your doctor and an aromatherapy professional. You may be surprised to find you can use aromatherapy in conjunction with or in lieu of some modern medicines. One thing's for certain—in the right hands, essential oils are a powerful tool that can be used for a large number of therapeutic reasons.

Here are just some of the many therapeutic qualities essential oils can have:

- Antibacterial.
- Antifungal.
- Anti-inflammatory.
- Antimicrobial.
- Antioxidant.
- Antiparasitic.
- Antiseptic.
- Antispasmodic.
- Antiviral.
- Boosts immune system.
- Calming.
- Decongestant.
- Improved circulation.
- Improved digestion.
- Improved mental health.

- Improved organ function.
- Moisturizing of skin.
- Pain relief.
- Relaxing.
- Skin care.
- Skin healing.
- Stimulating.
- Wards off cancer.
- Well-being.

The best part about essential oils is that a single oil can feature a number of these benefits and you can combine oils to create interesting blends that smell great and have a even wider range of health benefits. There are literally hundreds of oils on the market, and there's the potential of creating hundreds of thousands of various blends with different qualities. The possibilities are endless.

A Brief History of Aromatherapy

While the terms "aromatherapy" and "essential oil" are relatively new, the use of plant oils to improve health been around in one form or another for thousands of years.

The first documented use of plant oils dates as far back as 6,000 to 7,000 B.C. when our ancient ancestors discovered they could mix plant oils with animal fat and use it to heal illnesses, treat wounds and soothe the mind after a hard day of hunting and gathering. While most modern films depict cavemen as stinky Neanderthals, the reality is they may have smelled pretty good from the plant oils they were mixing with fat and constantly rubbing onto their bodies.

As man evolved, so did the oils being used and the methods used to extract them. Instead of simply adding organic matter to animal fat and cooking it until the oils were extracted, distillation and pressing methods were discovered that allowed for the collection of large amounts of concentrated oils with powerful scents and even stronger healing properties. These oils were highly-sought after and it wasn't uncommon for ships to sail across the globe to gain access to treasured oils like sandalwood, frankincense, myrrh and patchouli.

Fleets of ships traversed the high seas to gain access to oils not otherwise available at home and trade agreements worth millions in today's money were made between nations. It isn't known for sure that essential oils were the first products traded for on a mass scale between nations, but some of the first documented trades involved large amounts of myrrh, cypress and other oils.

Because the logistics of traveling over land were too much to overcome, overseas trade routes that lasted for thousands of years were established. Egyptians, Romans and Europeans all traveled these trade routes to get access to the oils available in the Middle East, the Orient and even Africa. A large portion of the exploration of the world was done by explorers like Marco Polo and Christopher Columbus, who traveled the globe looking for shorter routes to distant lands where they could trade for exotic spices and oils.

Essential oils soon spread across the globe. They were used by everyone from kings and queens to the working poor. Religions soon adopted essential oils because of their spiritual qualities, further cementing them into popular culture. The use of essential oils for religious rituals is deeply ingrained into almost every religion across the globe. If they don't currently use essential oils, chances are they did at one time. None other than the Bible mentions a number of essential oils by name. Essential oils like frankincense and myrrh are well-known to this day because they were gifts given to Christ by the wise men when they traveled to see him from afar. Healing oils are also addressed in the Bible, which leads many of those who are religious to believe that God himself provided essential oils for our use.

Essential oils provided the first and most crucial link between the East and the West, and as a result, more than just fragrances were exchanged. Technology improved on both sides of the fence as different cultures adopted and improved upon ideas and inventions brought to them by foreign traders.

Aromatherapy started with the boiling of animal fat and plants to create the crude scented predecessors to modern massage oils. Plants and herbs were often burned to purify and add fragrance to the air. This eventually led to the creation of incense, which was formed by mixing plant matter with something that would cause it gum up and harden. Incense soon became immensely popular because it was easy to use and transport. As it spread across the globe, it was used for everything from air purification to warding off evil spirits. Back then, it wasn't just burned like it is today. It was rubbed into the skin, consumed as a dietary staple and added to baths and saunas.

As the popularity of incense rose, so did the use of plant oils. The Egyptians created oils so powerful the tombs of ancient kings contain pots that still have traces of the scent the oils they used to hold. Oils become popular components of perfumes and were used to make people smell and feel good at the same time. Massage oils became popular as people mixed and matched oils and rubbed them into their muscles to ease pain and relieve tension. Oils were ingested to help with digestive problems, headaches and stress. Over the ages, tens of thousands of uses for essential oils have been discovered, covering everything from dry skin to inability to perform in bed. While the science behind them wasn't understood until recently, what people did realize was that they worked to treat a number of illnesses and ailments. For centuries, essential oils were the go-to medicine for a number of cultures across the globe.

It wasn't until the last century or so that the use of essential oils began to separate from medicine. The rise in popularity of synthetic perfumes with no health benefits was the biggest separating factor, as people began to view fragrances as simply something that smelled good, but had no health value. Modern medicines gained popularity in leaps and bounds as synthetic chemicals were brought to market claiming to cure anything and everything. While many of the original medicines didn't work as advertised, they pushed holistic medicine to the brink of extinction as the civilized world turned to Western medicine to cure their woes.

Fast forward to the late 1920's and a man named Rene-Maurice Gattefosse "discovered" the healing benefits of essential oils when he burned his hand and dipped it in lavender essential oil to ease the pain. The quick recovery time from his injury led to the rediscovery of essential oils as a therapeutic agent. Gattefosse coined the term aromatherapie, and went on to publish a number of books about the benefits of essential oils. Driven by his experimentation (and that of others who soon joined the cause), plant oils slowly but surely made their way back into the limelight, albeit not at the same level of popularity they'd previously enjoyed.

In the last decade or so, essential oils have seen a revival as people look for alternatives to Western medicine. Modern practitioners of aromatherapy use essential oils to improve the health of their patients naturally. Those people in the know are quickly coming to realize modern medicine may not be all it's cracked up to be. More and more people are looking for holistic and natural means to rebalance their bodies as nature intended instead of using chemicals that further unbalance the human body's delicate chemical composition.

How Essential Oils Are Used

Essential oils are delivered to the body in one of three ways: through the nose and lungs, through the skin or through the digestive system. You have to inhale their fragrance, consume the oil or apply the oil topically to reap their benefits. In order to get the most from your essential oils, you need to be able to deliver them to your body in a manner that doesn't change the chemical composition of the oil and will net you the maximum health benefit from your oils. The good news is there are a wide variety of methods you can employ to do this.

Before we get into the various ways you can use essential oils, I want to make something painfully clear. There are some oils that aren't going to lend themselves well to particular applications. Some oils are too harsh to be inhaled, some are too "hot" to be applied topically, and there are a number of oils that should never, and I mean never, be ingested. You need to research the oils you're planning on using to find out the best applications for those particular oils. Making a mistake can degrade your health instead of improving it.

Essential oils work best when used in small amounts. When adding a new oil to your bag of tricks, always dilute the oil heavily and test it in an inconspicuous area before using it on a larger area. You're much better off finding out you're allergic to an oil when you've only used a small amount, as opposed to slathering massage oil all over your body and suffering a wide-scale negative reaction.

For aromatherapy purposes, essential oils should not be consumed. Ingesting essential oils is the least effective method of delivering them because they have to pass through your digestive system on their way to the rest of your body. The strong acids in your stomach can damage the chemical constituents of the oil and dull or completely eliminate the health benefits you would have reaped had the oil been applied in another manner. There are a select few applications where ingesting an oil is preferable to applying it topically or diffusing it, but those applications are few and far between. An example of this would be oil that's ingested to help with digestion or stomach ache. Never take an oil or oil blend orally without first consulting with your doctor. Taking essential oils orally is beyond the scope of aromatherapy applications.

Topical Application

When you topically apply an essential oil, you deliver it to your body by applying it directly to the skin. This is usually done by diluting the oil with a carrier oil first, but there are times when weaker oils are used at full strength. Let's take a look at some of ways you can apply essential oils topically.

Direct Application (Neat)

This is the most dangerous form of topical application because it involves applying essential oil directly to the skin at full strength. Direct application is referred to as neat application in some literature.

Neat application should be avoided for all but the weakest of oils. If you have a reaction that sensitizes your skin, you may find your body rejects that oil every time it comes in contact with it after that, regardless of how much you dilute it before applying it. Skin rashes, itching, burning and a number of other problems can occur when your body reacts negatively to a neat application of essential oil.

The stakes are pretty high, so always consult with your doctor and an aromatherapy practitioner before applying an oil neat. There are a number of websites and books that list oils they say can safely be applied neat that aren't safe at all. Sure, most people may never have a reaction, but if you're one of the select few who do, you may pay a steep price.

I've seen a few websites touting a method of neat application called the Raindrop method, which involves dripping a number of drops of various oils up and down the spine and letting them soak in. This is a potentially dangerous method of delivery because you end up applying quite a bit of oil to the skin undiluted. This drastically ups your chance of having a negative reaction.

Massage Oil

Essential oils can be diluted with carrier oil and massaged into to the skin. Carrier oils are oils made from vegetable or animal fat that aren't as strong as essential oils. These oils don't have the same strength that essential oils do, but they're generally considered healthy oils that can be used to enhance essential oils and dilute them to the point that they can safely be applied topically.

The ratio at which you should blend your carrier oils and essential oils varies depending on the strength of the oils you're using, but a general rule of thumb is to mix between 3 to 6 drops of essential oil into a tablespoon of carrier oil. Keep it on the low end at first until you test your skin to see if it is sensitive to the oils you're using. If you plan on applying the blend to sensitive areas like the face, dilute it even more. Start off using a drop or two of oil and test to see what happens. You can always add a little bit more later on if you don't get the desired effect.

Direct Application (Diluted)

You can dilute your essential oil with carrier oil and apply it directly to the skin without massaging it in. Pick an area and gently rub the oil blend into your skin. It should absorb rather quickly, leaving behind a protective coating on your skin. Some people don't like this coating and say it leaves their skin feeling oily or greasy. Other people love it because they feel like it protects their delicate skin from the harsh elements.

Bath Time

Essential oils can be added to your bath water to create a warm, relaxing bath experience that leaves your mind feeling invigorated and your body and skin feeling renewed. You can use stimulating oils in the morning to help you wake up and prepare for the day. Switch over to sedative or relaxing oils in the evening in order to wind down before bed.

For best results, add 5 to 10 total drops of oil to your bath water as you're filling the tub. Keep the harsher oils to less than three drops and combine oils with similar qualities. An example of this would be to add a few drops each of lavender and Roman chamomile to your tub at the end of the day to help you relax.

You can also add a few drops of your favorite oil to a footbath and soak your feet in it for a while. You shouldn't add more than 4 or 5 drops of oil to a footbath. Make sure you use relaxing oils and steer clear of oils that can irritate the skin.

Compress

Fill your sink up with hot or cold water. You want it to be as hot or as cold as you can stand it. Add a few drops of essential oil to the water and stir it up. Let the oil rise to the top of the water and use a folded towel to soak it up. Apply the compress to sore muscles or to the area of your body that you want to benefit most from the compress. Avoid sensitive area like your face and neck and be sure not to get any of the oil-infused water into your eyes. Leave the compress on for up to 45 minutes. If any irritation occurs, remove the compress and wipe away excess oil.

Create Your Own Product

This method takes a lot more effort than the others, but it can be rewarding to create skin care products and lotions that are tailor-made to your body and skin type. Take a base cream or lotion and add a few drops of your favorite essential oils to it. You can make face creams, skin creams, lotions, salves and all sorts of other products once you understand what the various essential oils are used for.

Inhalation

Inhalation of the fragrances of essential oils is a powerful way to deliver the health benefits of essential oils to your body. When you inhale essential oils, the molecules enter directly into your blood stream and are rapidly spread throughout your body. In addition to entering your bloodstream, they interact with your brain when they reach the olfactory nerves in your nasal cavity.

There are a number of means through which you can inhale the fragrances. Hot methods, in which you heat the oils to disperse them into a room, are generally considered to be less effective than cold methods because heating the oils can change their chemical composition. We're going to cover both hot and cold methods in this section.

Direct Inhalation

Direct inhalation takes place when you inhale the undiluted fragrance of an essential oil. The following methods of direct inhalation are commonly used:

- Add a few drops of oil to a napkin or a handkerchief and hold it over your nose. Breathe deeply.
- Apply a small amount of diluted oil to your upper lip. Inhale deeply.
- Rub a few drops of a weaker oil between your palms. Cup your hands and place them over your nose and mouth. Inhale the fragrance deeply.
- Take the cap off of the bottle containing the oil. Lift it to within a couple inches of your nose and breathe in the aroma.

- Fill your sink with hot water. Add 5 to 10 drops of oils to the water. Place a towel over your head, hold your face over the sink and inhale the steam.

Diffusion

Essential oils can be diffused into a room for a longer-lasting effect. Diffusers vaporize the oil and disperse tiny molecules of oil throughout the room. They can be used to purify the air and for therapeutic purposes. The best part is everyone in the room gets to enjoy the benefits and the good smells.

There are literally hundreds of types of diffusers on the market. Some use heat, which we've already discussed as not being ideal for essential oil diffusion. Others use cool air, which is the preferred method of delivery whenever possible. Here are some of the hot methods of diffusing essential oils:

- **Candle diffusers.**
- **Diffusers that heat up wax cubes, like the Scentsy warmers.**
- **Diffusers that use the heat of a light bulb.**
- **Electric diffusers that have a heating element.**
- **Incense that is infused with oils that's burned to release the scent.**

While it's known that these methods aren't ideal, they're still in use. Many people don't know that heat can negatively impact essential oils. Others know, but aren't all that concerned with the health benefits of the oils they're using and are simply using them to make the room they're diffusing oils into smell good.

Cold diffusion methods are generally considered to be more effective because they don't heat the oil before dispersing the fragrance into the room. The following methods are used to disperse oil without heating it:

- **A cotton ball soaked with oil, then placed in a small bowl can effectively disperse fragrance throughout a small room.**
- **Atomizers and nebulizers turn oils into a fine mist that is dispersed into the room.** If you use this method, only use it for a few minutes at a time. Large amounts of oil are dispersed very quickly and you don't want to waste oil or irritate your mucous membranes. This method works well in larger rooms and in situations in which you want more oil to be dispersed into the air.
- **Fan diffusers blow cool air across a reservoir containing essential oils mixed with water.** The fragrance is blown out into the room.
- **Reed diffusers use pots of oil into which long wooden sticks are placed.** The oil travels up the sticks and the scent is dispersed into the room.
- **Terra cotta pots are filled with oil and then a lid is placed on them.** The oil slowly seeps through the porous material and disperses into the room.
- **You can add up to 10 drops of essential oil to a spray bottle full of water and use it to spray a fine mist of oil into a room.**

Diffusing large amounts of essential oil into a room or spraying oil directly on painted surfaces can damage paint and make it start to crack and peel. Use your oil sparingly and never spray it on a painted surface.

Olfactory Fatigue

Have you ever been somewhere that smelled particularly good or bad and noticed that after a while you got used to the fragrance and couldn't smell it anymore? What happened is your body grew accustomed to the smell as a process called olfactory fatigue kicked in.

In order to understand olfactory fatigue, we need to go back to ancient times and look at what the sense of smell was used for then. Back then, smell was used to identify two basic things: food and danger. Primordial man needed to be able to smell something and instantly tell whether it was a threat, something to dine on or something to be ignored. All other scents just got in the way. When a scent that was neither food nor a threat made its way to the brain, the brain processed it and discarded it as unimportant so it could focus on new scents coming into the brain that might be more important.

Olfactory fatigue is the modern day version of the threat or food assessment. When you smell something for a prolonged period of time and don't give it priority, your brain assumes that the scent is unimportant and discards it. You become immune to that scent as long as you remain in the area. That's why workers are able to work in stinky sewers for long periods of time and farmers are able to live on farms that have large amounts of manure present. You smell the stench as you pass through the area, but the farmers and workers have been there so long they don't smell it anymore.

Leaving the area permeated by the scent and returning or removing the scent from the room and reissuing it will allow you to smell it again for a short period of time because your brain has to reprocess the scent a second time. Each time your brain processes a scent, it will be able to discard that scent as unimportant at a slightly faster clip the next time it presents itself. Before too long, the body becomes almost completely immune to the scent. The brain recognizes it and processes it immediately.

For this reason, essential oils should be used sparingly and only for brief periods of time. 5 to 10 minute bursts of scent are much more effective than permeating a room with scent for hours on end. If you're in a room and you realize you don't smell a fragrance anymore, don't automatically assume there isn't any more oil in the diffuser and add more. It could be that you've become immune to the scent due to olfactory fatigue. Leave the room for a half hour and come back. You might be surprised to find you can smell the oil again, at least for a short period of time.

Setting your electric diffusers on a timer will allow you at least some level of control of when oils are diffused into a room. This method works well for light oils that have top notes that don't stick around for very long. Some essential oils are heavy and tend to linger around a room for hours or even days after they've been dispersed. What can you do then? Simple. Disperse the oil into a room that you don't spend a lot of time in and go into that room for 20 to 30 minutes at a time when you feel you need the benefits of the oil. Switch the oils that you're using up from time to time to keep your brain guessing.

Measuring Essential Oils

There are so many different measurements used for essential oils that it can make your head spin. Ounces, milliliters, drops, etc. There is no standard measurement used across the board. This chapter is designed to help you take the guesswork out of measuring your oils.

The most common unit of measurement you'll see in recipes that use essential oils is the drop. The problem with using a drop to measure oil is that a drop could mean something different to one person than it does to another. One person might assume a drop comes from an eyedropper, while another may surmise a drop should come from a turkey baster. That would result in the two people getting wildly different (and potentially dangerous) results from their oil blends. Let's clear something up right here and now. A single drop of essential oil is generally thought of as a drop from a standard eyedropper. There may be slight differences in volume between individual drops, but not enough to matter when it comes to making all but the biggest batches of oil blends and products.

There is no standard weight for a single drop because essential oils have different densities and weigh different amounts. There can be anywhere from 20 to more than 50 drops per milliliter of oil. While you could spend hours meticulously calculating out oil amounts, it really isn't necessary. It's safe to assume that 20 drops of oil equals 1 mL and go from there. You can always add more essential oil to future recipes if the results aren't what you expected.

While drops are an acceptable method of measurement for whipping up small batches of oil blends and product, you're going to want an easier method of measurement when it comes to measuring out larger amounts of oil. Nobody wants to sit around and count out 1000 drops oil for a large batch. This is where milliliters, teaspoons and ounces all come into play. It's up to you which method of measurement you use. We'll cover them all in this chapter, since it isn't uncommon to find recipes that use any of the three.

Here's a handy chart you're going to want to keep around:

Unit of Measurement	Converts to
20 drops	1 milliliter (mL)
100 drops	1 teaspoon (tsp)
300 drops	1 tablespoon (tbsp)
600 drops	1 ounce (oz)
1 teaspoon (tsp)	5 milliliters (mL)
1 teaspoon (tsp)	1/6 ounce (oz)
3 teaspoons (tsp)	1 tablespoon (tbsp)
3 teaspoons (tsp)	1/2 ounce (oz)
6 teaspoons (tsp)	1 ounce (oz)
1 tablespoon (tbsp)	15 milliliters (mL)
1 tablespoon (tbsp)	1/2 ounce (oz)
2 tablespoons (tbsp.)	1 ounce (oz)
1/2 ounce (oz)	15 milliliters (mL)
1 ounce (oz)	30 milliliters (mL)

Keep in mind that some of these conversions are rounded or estimated for the sake of ease of use. You can figure out exact amounts if you want to, but it's rarely critical and most people use these guidelines for measurement when mixing up small batches of oil. The larger the batch of oil you make, the more it's going to matter whether or not you use exact measurements. For most people making essential oil blends at home for personal use, the provided chart is more than adequate.

For larger batches, you're going to want to weigh out your oils or measure them by volume to make sure your blends stay accurate. Anything above a few ounces should be carefully measured so you can ensure you're getting the right amount of oil in your blends. If you plan on weighing your oils, get a good weighing scale that's accurate to at least the nearest tenth of a gram. If you plan on measuring by volume, invest in some good beakers and pipettes that are marked off in the unit you plan on using.

When you're blending oils, you may come across recipes that call for percentages instead of actual units of measurement. If an oil or an oil blend calls for 5% dilution, you need to figure out what 5% of the amount of carrier oil you plan on using is and add that amount of essential oil. If you have 1 teaspoon of carrier oil, a 5% dilution would equate to approximately 5 drops of essential oil. If you have an ounce of carrier oil, a 5% dilution would equate to .05 of an ounce of essential oil, which is 30 drops.

The formula to figure out how much essential oil is needed is as follows:

The amount of carrier oil * The percentage of dilution

Convert the percentage to a decimal before multiplying. 5% would become .05.

Here's a chart that makes some of the conversions for you, just to get you started:

Amount of Carrier Oil	Dilution Percentage	Amount of Essential Oil to Use
1 teaspoon (tsp)	10%	10 drops
1 tablespoon (tbsp.)	10%	30 drops
1 ounce (oz)	10%	60 drops
1 teaspoon (tsp)	5%	5 drops
1 tablespoon (tbsp.)	5%	15 drops
1 ounce (oz)	5%	30 drops
1 teaspoon (tsp)	4%	4 drops
1 tablespoon (tbsp.)	4%	12 drops
1 ounce (oz)	4%	24 drops
1 teaspoon (tsp)	3%	3 drops
1 tablespoon (tbsp.)	3%	9 drops
1 ounce (oz)	3%	18 drops
1 teaspoon (tsp)	2%	2 drops
1 tablespoon (tbsp.)	2%	6 drops
1 ounce (oz)	2%	12 drops
1 teaspoon (tsp)	1%	1 drops
1 tablespoon (tbsp.)	1%	3 drops

1 ounce (oz)	1%	6 drops

When you're creating blends, the amount of drops is the total combined number of drops of all essential oils added to the blend. If you're making a blend that requires 10 drops of essential oil and you're using Roman chamomile and lavender, you'll have to split the number of drops of each oil up so there are no more than ten drops total. You could use 5 of each, 4 of one and 6 of another, 3 of one and 7 of another, and so on. Some recipes tell you how to split the oils up; some leave it up to you. A good rule of thumb is to use more of the weaker oils and only a drop or two of the stronger oils.

If you're using "hot" oils that are capable of burning or irritating the skin, you're going to need to keep your dilution rate low. Start off at a 1% percent dilution and test it to see whether your skin reacts to the stronger oil. If you're planning on applying a product or oil blend directly to your skin and leaving it on your skin, your best bet is to keep the dilution below 3%. Always dilute oil blends and products that are going to be applied to your face or other sensitive areas to less than 1%.

What Essential Oils Are Made Of

Hydrogen. Carbon. Oxygen. These three elements combine to form thousands of compounds found in essential oils.

A single essential oil can contain hundreds of different compounds that combine to give it a unique scent and its own set of therapeutic benefits. Plants that smell alike contain a number of the same compounds along with a few different compounds that give them their own scent. That's why citrus fruits have a similar scent, but the scents are unique enough that you can tell an orange apart from a lemon solely based on smell.

The chemical composition of an essential oil determines how it acts when it enters or is applied to the human body. Each individual compound acts on the body in a different way. Some are beneficial and help the body improve both internal and external functions. Some are inert and pass right through the body. Inert compounds aren't harmful in small amounts, but they can add a heavy load to internal organs that are tasked with filtering them out and eliminating them. A handful of compounds are harmful and can damage the body and skin.

It's important that you understand how an essential oil is going to act on the body before you use it because you run the risk of doing permanent damage if you use an oil incorrectly. The only way to understand how an oil is going to act on your body is to have at least a basic knowledge of its chemical composition. You have to know what's in it in order to figure out what the impact of using the oil will be.

Oils of the same type can contain varying proportions of chemical compounds based on when the plants they were derived from were harvested, how they were grown and the method used to distill the oils, amongst a number of other factors. The term chemotype is used to describe oils that come from the same plant, but are chemically different. A chemotype is a consistent variation in an essential oil's composition. If a company is able to create an oil under certain conditions that has a consistent chemical composition from batch to batch, it becomes a chemotype. A plant identified as a chemotype is going to have qualities that are different from other standard oils of the same type.

The term chemotype leads people to believe that the oil has been altered chemically to give it different properties, but that isn't the case. An essential oil chemotype is a natural variation in an oil; not one that's created in a laboratory setting.

Let's look at some of the chemical constituents found in essential oils.

Isoprenes

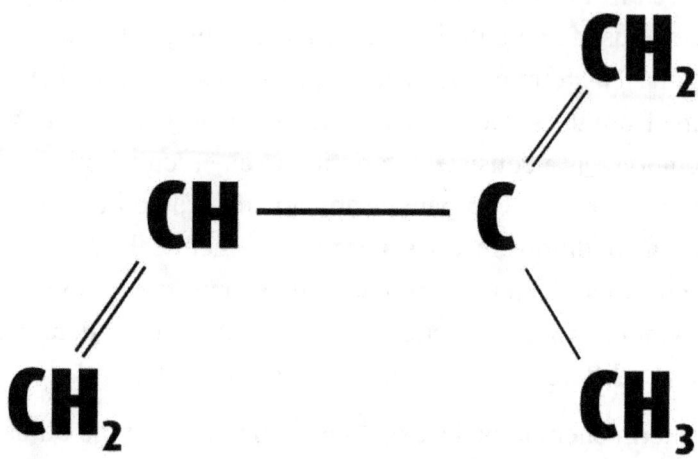

Figure 1: Basic isoterpene unit.

Isoprene units are the building blocks of essential oils. They are formed when 5 carbon atoms link up with 8 hydrogen atoms as shown in the picture above. Don't worry; you don't have to know the molecular structure of any of the compounds discussed in this chapter. I've just included them for those who are interested.

Think of isoprene units as little Lego pieces that can be snapped together to create a number of other types of molecules. Isoprene units link together to form compounds called terpenes.

Terpenes

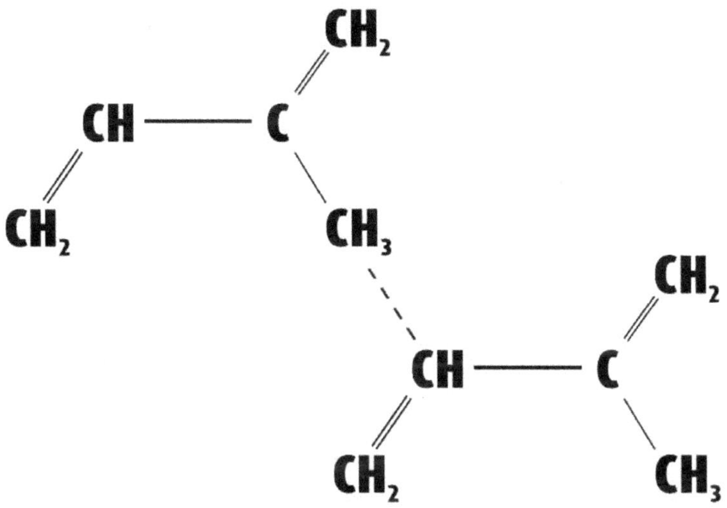

Figure 2: Monoterpene unit.

Terpene units are created when two isoprene units combine. The dotted line in the picture above shows where the isoprene units are connected. Terpenes can consist of anywhere from two isoprene units that are combined with a single link to thousands of isoprene units that are connected via multiple paths and chains.

Monoterpenes contain 1 terpene unit (2 isoprene units); sesquiterpenes contain 1 ½ terpene units (3 isoprene units); diterpenes contain 2 terpene units (4 isoprene units); triterpenes contain 3 terpene units (6 isoprene units); and tetraterpenes contain 4 terpene units (8 isoprene units). Terpenes can get very complex. A tetraterpene contains 40 carbon atoms and 64 hydrogen atoms. While this list of terpenes is only the tip of the iceberg when it comes to terpenes found in nature, these 5 terpene types are the only ones you need to be concerned with when it comes to essential oils. The bigger terpene molecules with more than 5 units generally don't make it through the distillation process. As a matter of fact, even diterpenes, triterpenes and tetraterpenes rarely make it through distillation. There may be trace amounts of them in your essential oil but they're rarely found in abundance.

There are literally thousands of different types of terpenes found in essential oils. Whenever you see an ingredient that ends in –ene, you're looking at a terpene of one form or another.

In addition to bonding with one another, terpene units can also bond with oxygen atoms, creating oxygenated terpene compounds. These terpenes go by a number of different names. We'll get to them later on in the chapter.

Monoterpenes

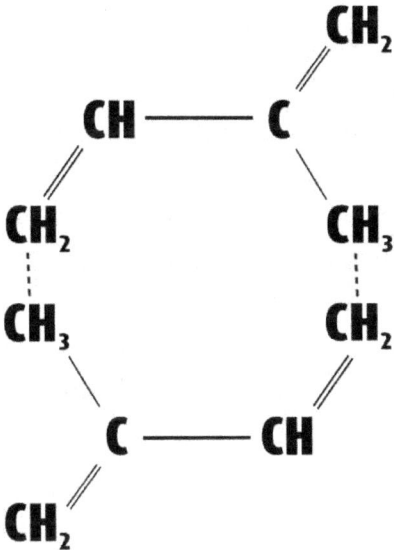

Figure 3: Monoterpene linked to form ring.

Monoterpenes are created when 2 isoprene units link together. They contain 16 hydrogen atoms and 10 carbon atoms. Figure 2 in the previous chapter shows a monoterpene unit in which the two isoprene units are linked together at a single location. The dotted line indicates the link between the units. Isoprene units can also link together to form what's known as rings. Figure 3 above shows a monoterpene with a ring created when isoprene units link together at multiple locations.

As many as a thousand different monoterpenes have been identified to date, many of which can be found in various amounts in essential oils. Since monoterpenes are the smallest terpene unit found in essential oils, they easily pass through the distillation and filtering process and are the most abundant component in essential oils. Monoterpenes are responsible in large part for the smell and flavor of a plant and its associated essential oil(s).

Monoterpenes are believed to have antiseptic, analgesic, decongestant, stimulant and antioxidant properties. These powerful compounds are able to rewrite DNA code into cells. Tests on animals have shown some monoterpenes may be effective at helping ward off cancer by reducing the formation of tumors and increasing the number of enzymes used by the body to remove toxins. Additional testing is underway to determine just how effective a tool monoterpenes may be.

Monoterpenes are present in large amounts in many essential oils. Two of the more common monoterpenes found in essential oils are limonene and pinene. Limonene is present in large amounts in citrus oils. Grapefruit, tangerine and orange essential oils have lemonine content in excess of 90%. Lemon oil has between 60% and 70% lemonine by volume. Limonene is thought to help clear up skin problems, tone the skin, aid with muscle stiffness and arthritis pain, aid with digestion and help with sore throats. It's also one of the monoterpenes currently being tested for its tumor fighting abilities.

Pinene comes in two forms: α-pinene and β-pinene. It's found in the oils of coniferous trees like pine trees, and in a number of other oils including lavender, eucalyptus, tea tree and rosemary oil. Pinenes have antifungal, anti-inflammatory, antimicrobial, antiviral, expectorant and insect repellent properties and the oils containing them can be used to treat respiratory conditions.

Angelica root oil is made up of nearly 90% monoterpenes. There are almost 30 different monoterpenes found in angelica root oil, including two types of pinene and limonene. Frankincense is another oil that's high in monoterpenes. It contains as high as 70% monoterpenes.

Sesquiterpenes

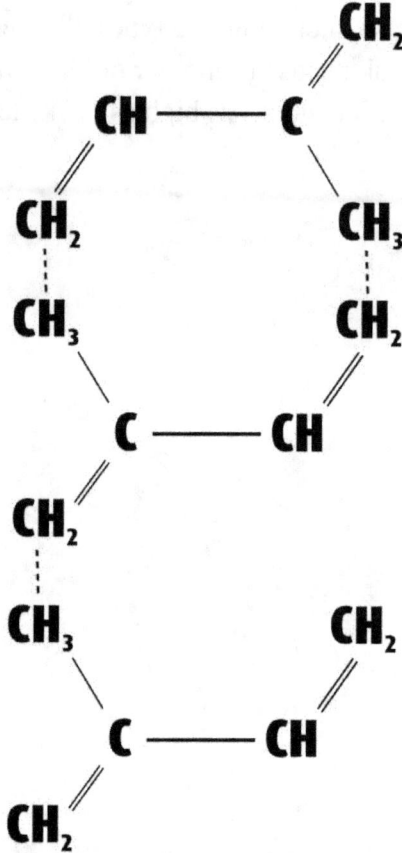

Figure 4: Sesquiterpene

Sesquiterepenes are formed when three isoprene units form a bond. They contain 24 hydrogen atoms and 15 carbon atoms. There are numerous ways that sesquiterpenes can bond. At least 10,000 different sesquiterpenes have been identified to date.

Sesquiterpenes act on cells by delivering oxygen molecules to them and deleting bad code in the cell. Once the bad code is deleted, monoterpenes take over and rewrite good code where the bad code previously was. Sesquiterpenes may also be able to fight cancer and studies are underway to determine how effective they are. In addition to the above qualities, sesquiterpenes are believed to be antibacterial, antiseptic, anti-inflammatory and stimulant by nature. They're able to cross the blood brain barrier and deliver oxygen directly to brain cells.

Essential oils that are high in sesquiterpenes include Cedarwood, Sandalwood, ginger, blue cypress, Vetiver, black pepper, patchouli and myrrh.

Alcohols

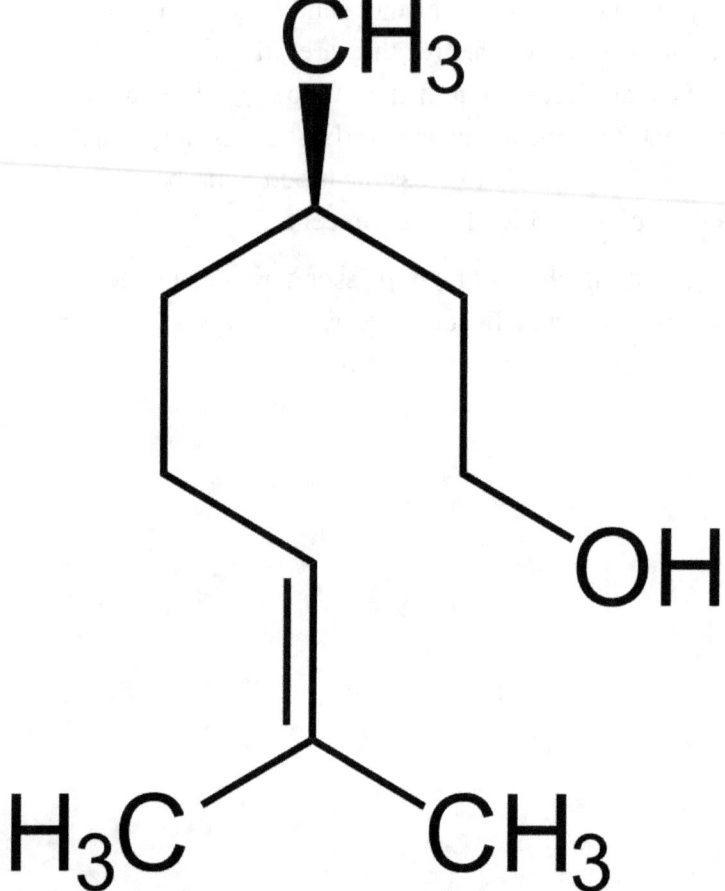

Figure 5: Citronellol molecule.

Alcohols are made up of convoluted combinations of carbon, hydrogen and oxygen molecules. They're created when OH radicals attach to other molecules.
Monoterpenols are created when an OH radical attaches itself to a monoterpene molecule. When an OH molecule attaches itself to a sesquiterpene, it creates a sesquiterpenol.

Alcohols can have antifungal, antiseptic, antibacterial, anti-infectious, anti-inflammatory, antiviral, diuretic and tonic capabilities. They're thought to stimulate the immune system and promote emotional well-being. They can also be used for skin care purposes and can promote healing of damaged skin. Some oils with alcohol compounds in them have a sedative effect and some can be used as a local anesthetic.

The names of alcohol compounds end in the letters –ol. Geraniol, menthol, linalool and citronellol are all alcohols that can be found in essential oils. Eucalyptus, cedarwood, patchouli, Vetiver, chamomile, geranium, lemon, rosewood and lavender oils are all known to contain alcohol compounds.

Phenols

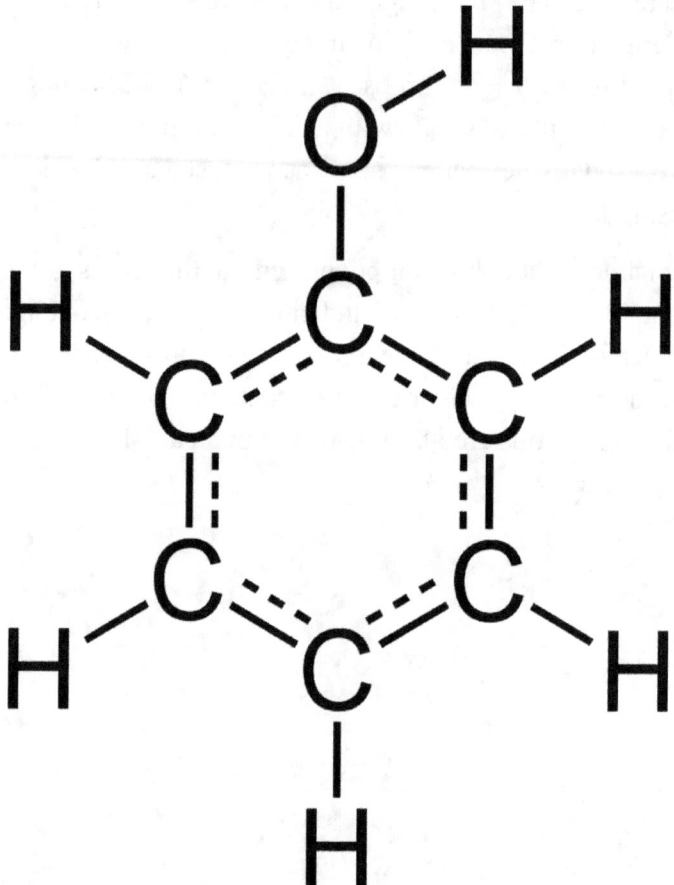

Figure 6: Phenol molecule.

Phenols are another powerful component of essential oils. Basic phenol molecules contain 6 carbon atoms and 6 hydrogen atoms in what's known as a benzene ring.

These oxygenated molecules cleanse cell receptors and have analgesic, antiseptic, antibacterial, anti-inflammatory, disinfectant, oxygenating and stimulant qualities. They combine with monoterpenes and sesquiterpenes to drive a powerful three-way cleansing and reprogramming of cells in the body.

The –ol at the end of phenol is indicative of an alcohol compound. Phenols are similar enough to alcohols that they're named in a similar manner, but they're different from alcohols in the manner in which they function. Common phenolic compounds include eugenol, thymol and carvacol.

Cinnamon, thyme, clove, oregano and savory essential oils all contain phenols. Use essential oils containing phenols with extreme caution, as they are known to be irritating to the skin. They place an added load on the liver and can irritate both the skin and mucous membranes. Always dilute them heavily and use them in small amounts for short durations of time. Test for a reaction prior to use.

Aldehydes

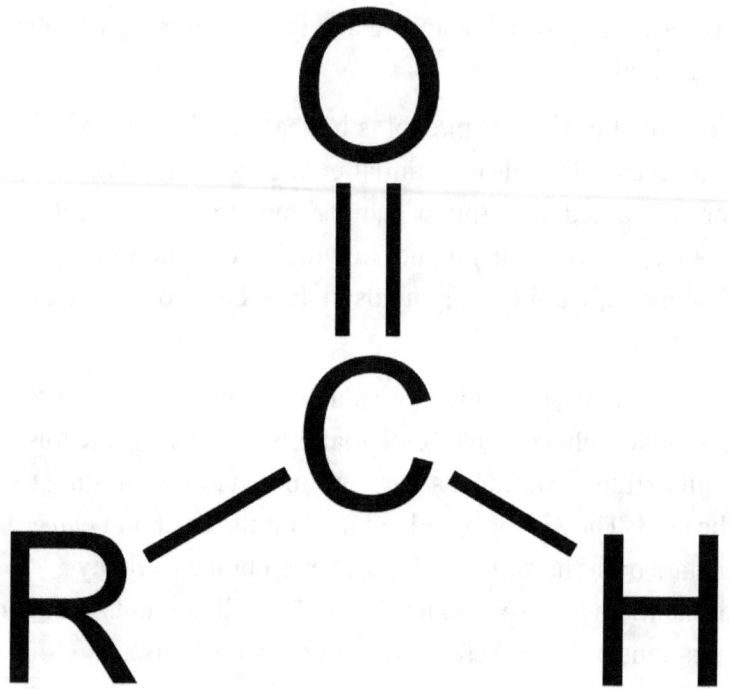

Figure 7: Basic molecular structure of an aldehyde.

Aldehydes are formed when a C=O grouping combines with a hydrogen (H) atom and a hydrocarbon group (R). There are at least a couple hundred different aldehydes found in essential oils. Aldehydes are easy to identify because they have names that end in –al or –aldehyde.

When aldehydes are present in essential oils, they contribute something unique and strong to the scent. They also have a strong flavor. If you've ever eaten cinnamon gum or candy, you've tasted cinnamal, which is one of the more distinctive aldehyde flavors. Vanillin aldehyde gives vanilla ice cream its unique aroma and flavor. Oils that are known to contain aldehydes include cinnamon bark, citronella, anise, cassia, lemongrass, lime, cumin, Roman chamomile, eucalyptus, onycha, thyme and vanilla. Most aldehydes have aromas that are highly sought after and enjoyed. The exception to this rule is valerian, which contains valeranal. This powerful aldehyde has a stench that most people can't stand.

Along with their powerful smell and taste, aldehydes also pack a potent punch. They're anti-infectious, antibacterial, anti-inflammatory, antispasmodic, antiviral, tonic, calming, relaxing and aphrodisiac by nature. They can help lower blood pressure and have been used to help reduce fevers.

Some aldehydes can act as a skin and mucous membrane irritant. Citral, found in citrus oils, is a strong irritant on its own, but isn't as strong when it's applied as part of an oil. Combining oils with aldehydes with oils high in terpenols can cool them down a bit and will make them more tolerable to the skin. It's still a good idea to use them with caution and always test on a small area prior to application. Some people have strong negative reactions to aldehydes regardless of how they're blended. Oxidized aldehydes are especially problematic, so store your essential oils that have aldehydes in them in a dark bottle in a cool, dark place.

Esters

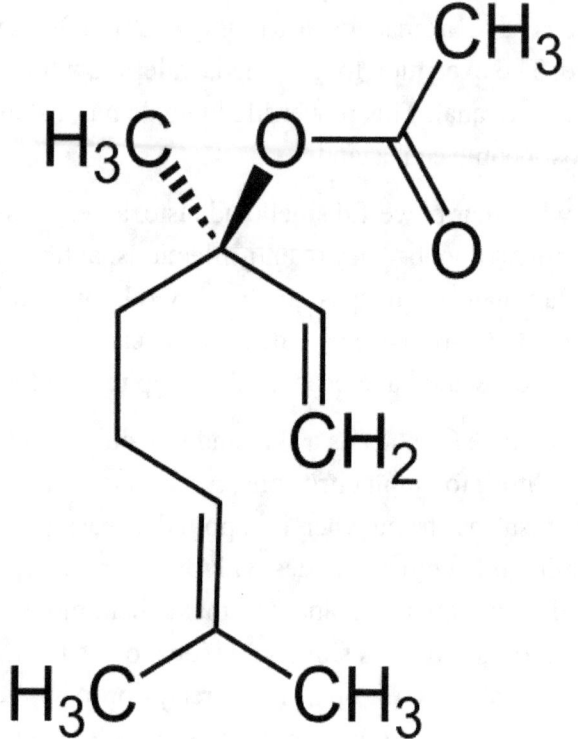

Figure 8: Linalyl acetate.

Esters are complex compounds formed when alcohols combine with acids to form new chemical compounds. The acid is usually completely removed from the oil when the reaction that forms esters takes place. There will still be some of the alcohol left. Esters generally add a fruity smell to the oils they're in.

Esters are named after the alcohol and the acid they were formed from. The –ol at the end of the alcohol's name changes to –yl and the –ic at the end of the name of the acid becomes –ate. Linalyl acetate, shown in the picture above, is formed when acetic acid reacts with linalol to create a new compound. Linalyl acetate is found in lavender essential oil. Other oils that contain high levels of acetates include bergamot, birch, cardamom, clary sage, geranium, helichrysum, lavender, myrtle, myrrh, petitgrain, Roman chamomile, ylang ylang and wintergreen. Most oils have at least small amounts of esters in them.

The esters in essential oils are generally considered safe for most aromatherapy applications. They are calming and balancing, anti-inflammatory, antiviral, antifungal, antispasmodic, sedative, soothing, and uplifting. Some esters are also analgesic.

Ethers

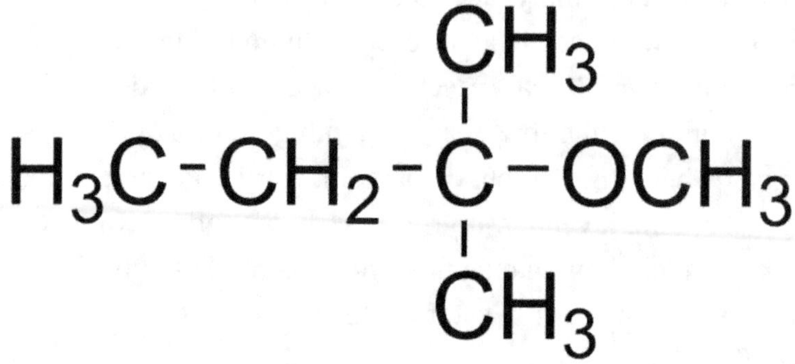

$$H_3C-CH_2-\underset{\underset{CH_3}{|}}{\overset{\overset{CH_3}{|}}{C}}-OCH_3$$

Figure 9: Amyl methyl ether.

Ethers are complicated molecules that aren't as common as many of the other compounds, but can have profound effects on taste, smell and therapeutic benefits when they're present. They can also be extremely toxic, so be sure to consult with your doctor and an aromatherapy professional before using oils containing them.

There is no naming convention for ethers. Some of the ethers you may come across in essential oils include asarone, cinnamaldehyde, eugenol methyl ether, methyl chavicol and safrole. They are found in aniseed, apiole, cinnamon bark, fennel seed and tarragon oil.

Essential oils containing ethers are powerful oils that should be used with caution. They are antispasmodic, sedative and anesthetic by nature. Many aromatherapists avoid oils like parsley seed, boldo and calamus that have high ether content because of their toxicity. Heavily dilute oils containing ethers and only use them for short periods of time because they can be neurotoxic and can be dermal irritants.

Some ethers may be carcinogenic. Asarone in particular has been shown to promote the growth of tumors in lab testing on animals.

Ketones

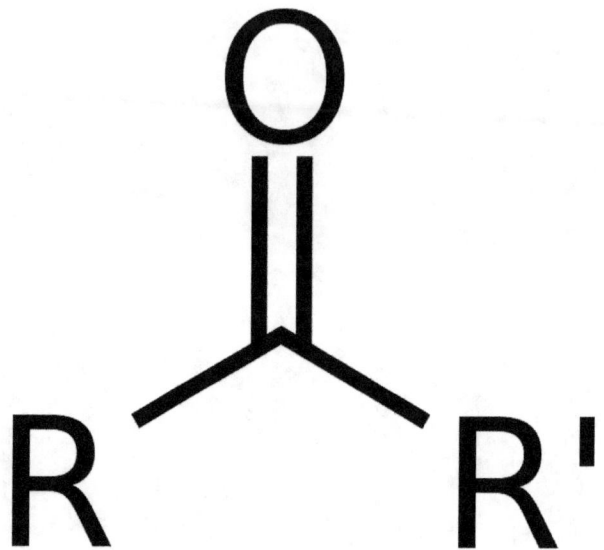

Figure 10: Ketone grouping.

Ketones feature two carbon atoms bonded to a carbonyl group. They're a relatively rare occurrence in essential oils, but the oils that have them tend to be extremely powerful. Tiny amounts of ketones in an oil can have a significant effect on its taste and fragrance. The names of ketones generally end in –one. One notable exception is camphor, which is found in rosemary oil.

Many ketones are neurotoxic and should not be used for extended periods of time. Thujone is one of the strongest ketones and should generally be avoided for aromatherapy purposes. There is some literature that indicates sage oil has the ability to quench at least some of the harmful effects of the thujone it contains, but it should still only be used under the supervision of an aromatherapy professional and with the approval of your doctor. Menthone, pinocamphene and pulegone are other ketones that are found in essential oils that are generally avoided. If you do decide to use oils that have these ketones, proceed with extreme caution. Dilute them to less than 1% and only use them for short periods of time.

Found in basil, coriander, rosemary, lemon eucalyptus, thyme and white camphor essential oils, camphor is one ketone aromatherapists usually love. Camphor is one of the main active ingredients in Vicks Vapor Rub. Believe it or not, there is anecdotal evidence that indicates inhaling camphor may create cravings that border on addiction in some people. It can be toxic in larger amounts and should never be taken internally, but does have its external applications. It has a narcotic and sedative effect and is also used as a decongestant. It's also used to relieve minor muscle aches and pains.

Eucalyptus, hyssop, peppermint and rosemary oils all have small amounts of ketones in them. These oils are generally considered to be safe for use, but should be used with caution and only in small amounts. The health benefits of the lesser-toxic ketones include antibacterial, antifungal, antispasmodic and regenerative properties. They're used to regenerate damaged skin and tissue and have mucolytic effects that can help with congestion.

Lactones

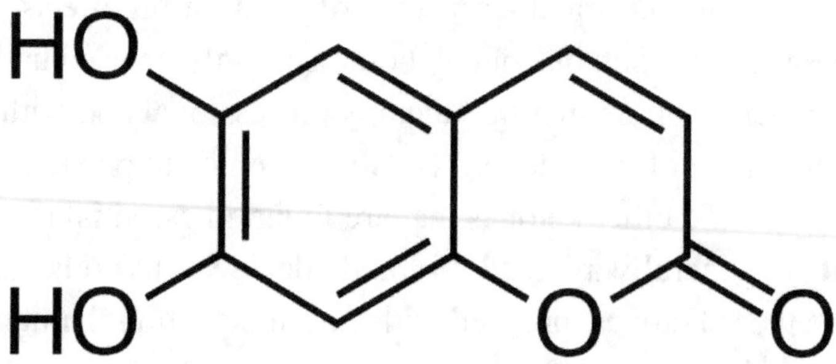

Figure 11: Aesculetin (lactone found in peppermint).

Lactones are similar in form and function to ketones, except that the single-bonded oxygen atom is part of a hydrocarbon ring. They are created from molecules that contain both acid and alcohol radicals. There is no naming convention for lactones. You may see some that end with – lactone, but they are few and far between.

Anise, catnip, lime, lavender and Roman chamomile oils all contain lactones. They have expectorant properties and can be used to relieve congestion. They're also antiseptic, antispasmodic and anti-inflammatory. Be careful when using oils that contain lactones because they can cause sensitization issues and they're phototoxic, meaning they make the skin more sensitive to the sun than it usually is.

Oxides

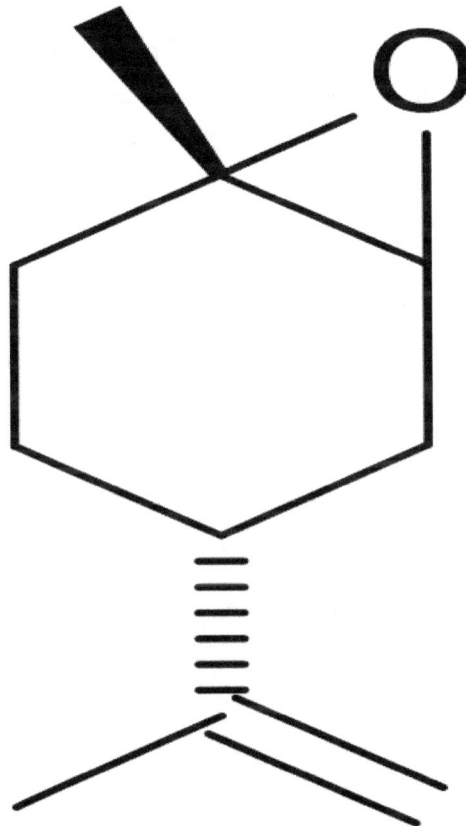

Figure 12: Limonene oxide.

Oxides form from the other compounds found in essential oils when they oxidize. Oxidation happens when an oxygen atom attaches to 2 carbon atoms of the same molecule. Oxides are usually denoted by adding the word oxide after the original compound. Limonene becomes limonene oxide when it oxidizes.

Cajeput, carrot seed, eucalyptus, German chamomile, peppermint and ravensara essential oils all contain large amounts of oxides. Eucalyptol, also known as cineole or cajuputol, is an oxide found in most essential oils in at least trace amounts. Eucalyptus, cajuput and black peppermint oils all have levels of eucalyptol in excess of 60%. Cineole has antiseptic, stimulant and expectorant qualities. They can be toxic in large amounts, so keep your blends to less than 2%.

Essential Oil Quality

It's tough to judge the quality of an individual essential oil because there are no government or organizational standards by which oils are judged. What one company deems to be high quality oil may be substandard in the eyes of another. Most companies don't publish the standards by which they judge their oils, so there's no easy way to tell what's in an oil before you buy it. When in doubt, it doesn't hurt to ask. Just be aware that you may not be getting the full story. There are unscrupulous companies out there that misrepresent and even mislabel the oils they sell to maximize profits.

While most literature says to use only therapeutic grade essential oil for aromatherapy purposes, the term "therapeutic grade" is largely left up to interpretation. One could easily surmise from reading this term that it means the oil is of a high quality, but that may not always be the case. Instead of blindly trusting therapeutic grade oil is of the highest quality, it's important you actually verify this is true. The reality is most companies making claims they're selling "therapeutic" or "aromatherapy" grade oils are only making the claim because they know it'll help boost sales. Their oil may not be any better than that from the companies who don't make this claim—and in some cases the quality is far worse.

Only the highest quality oils should be used for aromatherapy. This means sourcing oils that are distilled using strictly controlled standards in order to ensure the oils remain pure and consistent in their chemical composure from batch to batch. There are a ton of variables that can affect the quality of essential oil and a reputable company will seek to standardize as many of those variables as possible. Strict control results in higher quality oil, but it also means the company selling the oil is able to charge a premium.

True top grade oils will have the following qualities:

- **The plants the oils are derived from will be grown in the right environment.** Quality plants are grown in the correct location and in the correct soil. The climate needs to be ideal in order for the plant to produce the best essential oils.
- **The plants will be grown at the correct altitude.** Growing plants at too high or too low of an altitude can affect the quality of the oil.
- **The plants should be grown organically.** It may be difficult to find organic oils for some of the rarer oil types. This factor shouldn't preclude you from using an oil when an organic version isn't available, but it's best to use organic oils whenever possible.
- **Plants must be harvested properly and stored in a manner conducive to harvesting the oils at a later time.** For most plants, it's best to harvest their oils when the plant is fresh. Allowing the plants to sit for long periods of time will impact the quality of oil you're able to get from those plants.
- **The correct variety of plant needs to be used.** Essential oils like lavender can be distilled from different varieties of lavender. English, Bulgarian and French lavender plants (amongst others) can all

be used to make oil that's labeled as lavender essential oil. Some varieties of plants make better oils than others. Reputable suppliers will list what variety of plants their oils are derived from and what country they're sourced from. It's up to you to do the proper research to determine which plants make the best oils.

- **The part of the plant that the oil is distilled from makes a difference in quality as well.** Oils distilled from seeds or pods will have different qualities than oils distilled from hardwood, stems, leaves or roots. Again, the supplier should indicate what part of the plant their oil is extracted from.

- **The method of distillation should be the best method for that particular plant.** Some plants lend themselves well to different types of distillation. An oil distilled through use of steam will have different qualities than one extracted through use of CO_2. Again, it's important to know which methods work best for a particular oil.

- **Chemicals and solvents should be avoided whenever possible.** While there are some oils that have to be extracted using solvents, you should avoid oils distilled in this manner whenever possible because trace amounts of the solvent can be left behind.

- **Nothing should be added to the oil after extraction.** No dilution of the oil or adding of synthetic chemicals should take place. High quality essential oils should be able to stand on their own two feet without need to supplement them with anything else. The exception to this rule is when extremely expensive oils are adulterated with less expensive oils in order to make them more affordable to the average buyer. When this takes place, a reputable manufacturer will clearly label the oil as adulterated and will indicate what it's been adulterated with. This isn't done in an attempt to deceive. It's done in an attempt to moderate the cost.

- **Oils should be stored properly after distillation.** Essential oils need to be stored in a cool, dark place until they're bottled up and shipped out. The bottles should be dark. Clear glass bottles are a sign of a supplier that doesn't care about the quality of his oils.

When you're buying essential oils, it's rarely a good idea to search out the cheapest supplier you can find. These suppliers often take shortcuts that seriously damage the quality of their oils. There's no standard that they're held to, so they create budget oils that are of sub-par quality—and most people don't know the difference. One trick used by shady manufacturers is to mix cheaper oils to get them to smell like more expensive oils and then to sell them as the more expensive oil.

It's important that you only use pure oils that are unadulterated whenever possible. When manufacturers adulterate oils without notifying consumers, they often use substances that can put your health at risk instead of improving it. A supplier adding synthetic compounds to their oils to give it a similar scent as higher quality oil is never a good thing. Reputable manufacturers will label their oils when they've been adulterated, but this isn't always the case. Suppliers have been known to adulterate expensive oils with cheaper oils that have similar scents. This allows the supplier to sell the adulterated oil at the higher cost of the expensive oil. It's misleading and probably illegal, but there isn't anyone monitoring to see if it's happening. It's unknown just how widespread of a problem this is, but as with anything that's largely unmonitored, it's happening at least some of the time.

You may come across perfume grade oils in your search for a reputable supplier. These oils are made to be used in perfumes and have the scent of essential oils. They rarely have the same therapeutic qualities. People who make perfumes are largely concerned with the smell and rarely worry about health benefits. Synthetic fragrances are even worse. They're designed in a lab to smell good, but have no health benefit. In fact, they can cause problems because they tend to be harsh and are hard on the skin.

Food grade oils should also be avoided. They're manufactured to have a standard taste and smell and the manufacturers add or remove components to ensure they maintain that standard. You want pure oils, not oils that have been adjusted to meet some criteria set by a scientist in a lab.

In the previous chapter, we discussed the key chemical constituents of essential oils. The fragrance of these components can be faked through use of synthetic materials that mimic the organic components, but fall well short of the mark when it comes to health benefits. The good news is there are ways to test oils to make sure they're of a high quality. The bad news is many of these methods require specialized equipment that's expensive and hard to find. Gas chromatography (GC) can be used to identify the individual chemicals that make up an oil. This method uses a special machine that heats up the oil, causing it to evaporate. As it evaporates, it rises to the top of the machine and passes through a sensor that records when and how much liquid evaporated at each incremental increase in temperature. The temperature at which evaporation took place is used to determine what the constituents are. This method is highly accurate, but the machines cost thousands of dollars and aren't something the average aromatherapist is going to have on hand.

While the machines and the know-how to read the graph created by machines are beyond the means of most people, if you're really concerned with making sure your oil is of the highest quality, you could send it out to a lab to get tested. Ideally, you'd want to have a gas chromatography and mass spectrometry test run on it. This will determine what your oil contains and whether any adulterants have been added to it.

Or you could just go with a reputable supplier that has a proven track record. Your call.

Just remember this. When you're shopping around for oils and see an oil labeled as therapeutic or aromatherapy grade, the only entity judging the quality of that company's oil is the company itself. Your best bet is to seek out reputable companies that have been in business for a long time and are trusted by aromatherapists who are in the know. Even then, the quality could suffer a bit from batch to batch, but you'll generally be in good hands.

To get you started, I've gathered a list of some of the better-known and trusted companies selling oils today. I don't make any money off of you clicking these links. They're just provided to help you out:

http://www.100pureessentialoils.com/

http://www.amphora-retail.com/

http://www.anandaapothecary.com/

http://www.aqua-oleum.co.uk/

http://www.auroma.com/

http://www.camdengrey.com/

http://www.dropwise.com

http://www.elizabethvanburen.com

http://www.e-scent-ials.com/

http://www.fromnaturewithlove.com

http://www.gardenofessence.com/#!store

http://www.mountainroseherbs.com

You might have noticed DoTerra isn't on the list. While they may have decent quality oil that's thoroughly inspected, I have a tough time recommending a company that sells their products using multi-level marketing. For the same reason, I didn't add Young Living to the list. I will say this for both companies. There are a lot of people who swear by their oils. I personally can't attest to the quality of oils from either of these two companies, so I'll leave that decision up to you.

Cost vs. Quality

Aside from a handful of companies that rip people off by charging high prices for sup-par oils, you generally get what you pay for when it comes to essential oil. The price more often than not reflects the quality of the oil and the standards to which the company making the holds itself.

One thing you'll instantly notice is that some oils are infinitely more expensive than others. Some oils can be purchased for less than ten bucks an ounce, while others cost thousands of dollars an ounce.

The reason for this huge variance in price is the how difficult the oil is to obtain. One of the hardest oils to distill is jasmine, which requires almost 4 million jasmine blossoms per pound of oil. Contrast this with the less-expensive orange oil, which can easily be harvested from the peels of oranges, and you'll see why there's such a difference in price. At upwards of $400 an ounce, rose otto oil is another oil that demands a premium. It takes upwards of 5,000 blossoms to generate a pound of oil. That averages out to nearly 20 roses per single drop of oil. If you find either of these oils online for $30 an ounce, you should automatically know it's of poor quality and is full of synthetic additives.

Wood oils are anther oil type that's generally expensive because they have to be harvested from the hardwood of trees. The distillation of these oils requires that trees are grown to a certain size and/or age before they're harvested and harvesting them often means cutting them down to get to the valuable hardwood. Since trees can take decades or more to grow to the proper size, it can be difficult to keep up with the demand for popular hardwood oils. When you purchase hardwood oils, try to find oils from suppliers that use sustainable harvest methods or you may be contributing to the wholesale destruction of various species of tree.

Melissa oil is another oil that costs a small fortune. A pound of pure oil can cost as much as a small car. This sounds like a lot, and it is, but there's a good reason why the oil costs this much. It takes tons of Melissa plants to yield just a pound of Melissa oil. That's right, tons.

Steer clear of bargain basement oils. If it sounds too good to be true, it probably is. You aren't getting a great deal; you're getting a chemical cocktail filled with who knows what. Your local health food store or even your local big-box retailers like Wal-Mart and Target may have essential oils on sale for much less than what you see the specialty sites selling them for. That $10 bottle of frankincense oil isn't going to have the same health benefits that you'd get from buying the pure stuff online. The oil has more than likely been extracted using chemical solvents and/or high pressure distillation methods designed to harvest as much oil as possible from as many plants as possible in as short of a time as possible with little attention paid to the end-result. As long as it looks and smells like essential oil and is sold at the right price, people are willing to buy it—and most of the time they don't realize they aren't getting the health benefits.

If all you're concerned with is a good smell, then the budget oils might be passable. The smells usually aren't as smooth and tend to be sharper because of the additives, but the difference isn't all that noticeable to someone who hasn't smelled the real deal. On the other hand, if you're getting into aromatherapy because you want to reap the health benefits essential oils have to offer, you're going to be sorely disappointed by the discount oils that proliferate the market.

What I've found is spending a little extra actually saves money in the long run because pure oils that have been properly distilled are infinitely more powerful than the diluted budget oils. A bottle of pure oil lasts much longer than a bottle of junk oil because you won't have to use as much oil to get the same effect. You also won't have to worry about polluting your body with chemical additives that work against what you're trying to achieve by using the oils in the first place.

Essential oils are one area in life where you (usually) get what you pay for. Spend a little extra for the good stuff. You'll be glad you did.

Sustainability

Most people have no clue where in the world the essential oils they're buying are actually grown, harvested and distilled. As long as they're able to get their favorite oils, it's all too easy to turn a blind eye to whether or not the oils are coming from sustainable sources. This creates a system ripe for abuse, especially when you take into consideration the fact that many oils come from foreign countries where there is little to no oversight of the methods of harvest. Where there's a buck to be made, there are people willing to destroy entire forests and ecosystems to harvest plants that contain essential oils.

For this reason, it's important you ensure the companies you buy your oil from only deal with suppliers who practice sustainable harvest of the plants they use to make their oils. This is easy when it comes to oils that come from domesticated crops like lavender and citrus oils. The plants and trees these oils come from are easy to grow and are grown across the globe.

It gets a little more difficult when you're dealing with specialty oils that are confined to a handful of areas scattered across the globe. Sandalwood is one such oil. Sandalwood trees only grow in a few places, primarily in India and Australia. The oil is harvested from the heartwood of the Sandalwood tree. Traditionally, trees were harvested after 50 or more years of growth. This gives the heartwood plenty of time to grow and develop hardwood. Now, trees are being grown and harvested after 10 to 15 years because there are virtually no old growth trees left. The only old growth trees in existence are privately owned and have to be heavily guarded because armed criminals search them out and cut them down to get to their heartwood. This holds true for a number of wood oils. If a wood oil is harvested from hardwood, take a good, long look at the way it's harvested before you buy it. You may be contributing to the extinction of an entire species.

Any time an oil is labeled as coming from wild sources, your ears should perk up. Manufacturers use this term to indicate their oils are entirely organic and natural. The problem with wild sources is the wild plants may only grow in small areas. Pickers bounce from growth to growth harvesting everything in sight until there isn't anything left to harvest. Herb and spice oils are popular wild-harvested oils that are often harvested in a manner that isn't sustainable. Organic oils are great, but not if the cost is the wide-scale destruction of a plant species.

The manufacturer of the oil should be able to tell you whether or not their oils are harvested from sustainable sources. Don't assume just because a company is huge that it ensure sustainable sourced are used. Some of the biggest companies in the market are the worst offenders when it comes to sustainable harvesting.

Safety of Essential Oils

The tips in this chapter are general safety tips for essential oils. They don't take into consideration individual problems or concerns you may have. Always consult with your doctor before starting use of essential oils for aromatherapy purposes. If you're new to the world of essential oils, you should also enlist the help of an aromatherapy practitioner who can assist you in finding the correct blends of oils for your skin, your health condition and your body type.

It's important that you realize just how powerful essential oils are. Some oils contain the entire essence of a plant in just a drop or two of oil. Other oils contain the entire essence of multiple plants in just a few drops. A bottle of essential oil usually contains the oil from hundreds, if not thousands or tens of thousands, of plants. A little oil goes a long way. You don't want to use essential oils with the attitude that a little more won't hurt. A few drops more than what's recommended can be problematic. For some oils, more than a few drops extra can be toxic to both the skin and the internal organs.

You should store your essential oils where children can't access them. They smell good and young children may be tempted to play with them or even eat them. Even the weaker oils can wreak havoc on a young person's system in concentrated amounts. If you plan on using essential oils on your kids, only use oils your doctor says are OK and heavily dilute them before use. There are a handful of oils that are generally considered safe for use with children.

Your aromatherapy practitioner can help you identify the right oils and train you on how to properly apply them.

Be sure to read the labels on the essential oils that you're using to see if there are any special precautions. All oils are different and there may be considerations you have to make for that specific brand of oil, even if you've successfully used similar oils from other manufacturers.

If you're allergic to a particular type of plant or food, you're probably going to be allergic to its oil. You may also find you have a reaction to oils created in the same area as the oils that you're allergic to. When in doubt, contact the manufacturer to find out what oils are made in the same building as the oil you're buying.

When used properly and with care, essential oils are generally considered safe to use as long as you use them in the proper manner. There is a lot of misinformation out there regarding the safe use of these oils, so it's important to proceed with caution. Don't assume just because something worked for someone else that it's going to work in the same manner for you. Always test your oils in small amounts prior to using them to see how your body is going to react.

DANGER: Oils You Should Never Use

There are some essential oils that are too dangerous to use for aromatherapy purposes. The following oils should not be used for any purpose:

- **Alant root.** Powerful sensitizer.
- **Bitter almond.** Can contain cyanide.
- **Boldo leaf.** Can cause convulsion, even when used in small amounts.
- **Cade.** Strong sensitizer.
- **Calamus.** Contains the carcinogenic compound asarone.
- **Cassia.** Strong irritant of the skin and mucous membranes.
- **Yellow camphor (white camphor is OK, but should be used with caution).** Highly toxic when ingested.
- **Horseradish.** Strong irritant of the skin and mucous membranes.
- **Mugwort.** Toxic and can induce abortion.
- **Mustard.** Contains allyl isothiocyanate, which is unpleasant when inhaled and is a skin and mucous membrane irritant.
- **Pennyroyal.** Can induce abortion and is toxic to the internal organs, even in small amounts.
- **Rue.** Bad all the way around. It's neurotoxic, phototoxic and can damage the skin if applied topically. It can induce abortion as well.
- **Sassafras.** Contains safrole, a known carcinogen.

- **Tansy.** Contains thujone, which is a highly toxic compound.
- **Thuja.** Contains thujone, which is a highly toxic compound.
- **Wintergreen.** Strong skin irritant and toxic if ingested orally.
- **Wormseed.** Toxic to internal organs.
- **Wormwood.** Contains thujone, which is a highly toxic compound.

Note that this is not a complete list and there are other oils that exist that should not be used. The burden is on you to identify these oils. This list is just to get you started.

Contraindications

Be aware that if you have high blood pressure, diabetes, epilepsy or any other medical condition, you need to be careful when selecting essential oils for use. Let your doctor know about any oils you plan on taking well in advance, so he can help you identify potential problems before they occur. The rest of the chapter discusses some of the oils that need to be avoided if you have certain medical conditions. Don't assume that this is a complete list. It's not. There may be others not on the list that are every bit as dangerous. Always discuss any essential oils you plan on using with your doctor. You should also enlist the help of an aromatherapy practitioner when attempting to use essential oils safely when you have underlying medical conditions.

While there are women who use essential oils while pregnant to good results, you need to be very careful with what you use. The following oils should not be used by pregnant women:

- Angelica.
- Aniseed.
- Basil.
- Birch.
- Bitter almond.
- Calamus.
- Camphor.
- Cedarwood.
- Chamomile.
- Cinnamon.

- Clary sage.
- Clove bud.
- Fennel.
- Hyssop.
- Jasmine.
- Juniper berry.
- Marjoram.
- Mustard.
- Myrrh.
- Oregano.
- Peppermint.
- Rockrose.
- Rose.
- Rosemary.
- Sage.
- Tansy.
- Thuja.
- Thyme.
- Wintergreen.

Please note that just because an oil is on this list doesn't automatically mean it's safe to use while pregnant. To be completely honest with you, I'd recommend avoiding all but the most benign of essential oils while pregnant. Even then, I'd proceed with extreme caution and only do so under the supervision of a medical professional.

If you're epileptic or are otherwise prone to seizures, you need to avoid the following oils:

- Basil.
- Camphor.

- Eucalyptus.
- Fennel.
- Hyssop.
- Nutmeg.
- Pennyroyal.
- Rosemary.
- Sage.
- Spike lavender.
- Tansy.
- Thuja.
- Wormwood.

Some essential oils can influence your blood pressure. Those with high blood pressure need to avoid the following oils:

- Black pepper.
- Clove.
- Hyssop.
- Rosemary.
- Peppermint.
- Sage.
- Thyme.

Phototoxicity is a problem with certain oils. These oils need to be avoided if you're going to be exposed to sunlight for prolonged periods of time:

- Angelica root.
- Caraway.
- Cassia.
- Cinnamon bark.

- Citrus oils.
- Cumin.
- Dill.
- Ginger.
- Patchouli.
- Petitgrain.
- Rue.
- Verbena.

Carrier Oils

Most essential oils are too strong to apply topically at full strength. They tend to be on the "hot" side and can cause minor irritation or a reaction similar to a chemical burn when applied neat. Some oils are harsher than others and are more likely to result in irritation when applied at full strength. Your best bet is to assume all essential oils are too strong to apply neat and dilute them heavily. The level to which you need to dilute your oil depends largely on the oil itself and how harsh it is.

When in doubt, contact the supplier and find out what they recommend. Some oils are safe at 5% dilution, while others have to be diluted to 1% or less to be safe. You don't want to mess this up. Trust me.

Carrier oils, also known as base oils, are used to dilute essential oil. They come from the fatty portions of nuts, seeds and plants and are generally sold as food items. While carrier oils in and of themselves are generally considered safe to consume in small amounts, once you add essential oil, you change the carrier oil to the point where it may no longer be edible. Never consume carrier oil to which you've added essential oil without the express consent of your physician.

Carrier oils are used for the following reasons:

- **To dilute your essential oil and make it tolerable to the skin.**
- **To help essential oil penetrate deep into the skin.**

- **To stretch out expensive essential oils.** A few drops of essential oil in carrier oil will last a lot longer than trying to apply the essential oil undiluted.
- **To add therapeutic properties.** The carrier oils often have their own health benefits that they bring to the table.

When you buy carrier oil for aromatherapy purposes, seek out oils that have been cold-pressed. This is a process in which heavy stones or steel presses are used to grind and squeeze the carrier oil out of the plant matter they're derived from. Cold-pressed oils are some of the best oils you can buy because they haven't been heat-treated and aren't full of chemical additives and solvents.

Because they're derived from the fatty portions of plant, carrier oils can go rancid over time. If your carrier oil starts to smell rancid, it needs to be replaced. Essential oils don't have this problem, but they can oxidize and lose their health value.

Amino Acids in Carrier Oils

Amino acids are the building blocks the human body uses to create proteins. They link together to form the proteins the body needs to function and are responsible for every chemical reaction that takes place in the body. You can't live without a constant supply of amino acids.

There are 22 total amino acids that the body needs to function. There are 8 essential amino acids that you have to add to your body via your diet in order to ensure all 22 amino acids can be created. Here are the 8 essential amino acids that you have to consume because your body can't create them:

- Isoleucine.
- Leucine.
- Lysine.
- Methionine.
- Phenylalanine.
- Threonine.
- Tryptophan.
- Valine.

As long as you're adding these 8 amino acids to your body, the rest can be created.

There's a lot of confusion regarding amino acids in essential oils. Generally speaking, amino acids aren't present in essential oils in high enough amounts to be beneficial. While the plants that essential oils are made from contain amino acids, the oils derived from the plant rarely contain more than trace amounts.

Carrier oils, on the other hand, are derived from the fatty portions of plants and contain amino acids in large amounts. Using carrier oil as part of an oil blend allows you to add amino acids to your body when you apply the blend topically. The amino acids in carrier oil are readily absorbed into the skin.

Carrier Oil Information

The carrier oils in this chapter can be used for aromatherapy purposes. This section lists the following items about each carrier oil:

- **Price.** How expensive the oil is. Oils with a single $ are inexpensive, while oils with $$$$ command top dollar. $$ and $$$ indicate oils that fall somewhere in the middle.
- **Shelf life:** How long the oil typically lasts.
- **Scent:** What the oil smells like.
- **Color:** The color of the oil.
- **Source:** What part of the plant the oil is derived from.
- **Good for:** What the oil is good for.
- **Contains:** What nutrients the oil has in it.
- **Dilution:** Whether or not the carrier oil should be diluted or can be used at full strength.
- **Notes.** Additional information about the oil.

Sweet Almond Oil

Price:	$
Shelf life:	Up to 1 year.
Scent:	Sweet almond.
Color:	Light yellow.
Source:	Almond kernels.
Good for:	All types of skin. Softens and conditions skin. Leaves a slight residue.
Contains:	Oleic acid, linoleic acid, vitamins and minerals.
Dilution:	Used at 100% or as a blend with other carrier oils.
Notes:	Sweet almond oil is an inexpensive and popular choice when it comes to carrier oils. Do not use if you have nut allergies.

<u>Apricot Kernel Oil</u>

Price: $

Shelf life: Up to 2 years.

Scent: Nutty and slightly fruity.

Color: Light yellow to deep gold.

Source: Apricot seeds.

Good for: All types of skin. Especially good for dry or aged skin. Leaves an oily protective residue.

Contains: Oleic acid, linoleic acid, vitamins and minerals.

Dilution: Used at 100% or as a blend with other carrier oils.

Notes: Apricot kernel oil is similar to sweet almond oil and the two are often used interchangeably.

Andiroba Oil

Price:	$$ - $$$
Shelf life:	Up to 1 year.
Scent:	Musky and buttery.
Color:	Pale yellow.
Source:	Andiroba nuts.
Good for:	Damaged or injured skin. Used to ease the effects of eczema, psoriasis, cuts, burns and insect bites. Blends easily into the skin.
Contains:	Anti-inflammatory and insect repellent limonoids, oleic and linoleic acids.
Dilution:	Used at 100% or as a blend with other carrier oils.
Notes:	Andiroba oil is a thick liquid. It can be placed in warm water to make it more viscous and workable prior to adding essential oils.

<u>Argan Oil</u>

Price:	$$ - $$$
Shelf life:	Up to 1 year.
Scent:	Light and nutty.
Color:	Yellow.
Source:	Argan tree kernels.
Good for:	Dry skin. Used to hydrate skin and reduce stretch marks. Leaves slight residue.
Contains:	Oleic acid, linoleic acid, vitamins and minerals, phenols, tocopherols.
Dilution:	Used at 100% or as a blend with other carrier oils.
Notes:	Argan oil is one of the rarer carrier oils. It's highly-sought after because of its numerous health benefits.

Avocado Oil

Price:	$
Shelf life:	Up to 1 year.
Scent:	Sweet and nutty.
Color:	Deep green.
Source:	Avocadoes.
Good for:	All skin types, but works best on dry and damaged skin. Nourishes skin and hair. Leaves skin feeling waxy.
Contains:	Oleic acid, linoleic acid, vitamins and minerals.
Dilution:	Typically used at 5% to 10% of an oil blend or less.
Notes:	Avocado oil is a great additive oil that can be added to other carrier oils to add vitamins and minerals.

Borage Seed

Price:	$$ - $$$
Shelf life:	Up to 6 months.
Scent:	Sweet.
Color:	Pale yellow.
Source:	The seeds of the Borage plant.
Good for:	Most skin types, especially dry and damaged skin. Leaves oily residue after application.
Contains:	Oleic acid, linoleic acid, vitamins and minerals. Has higher levels of gamma linoleic acid (GLA) than any other oil.
Dilution:	Typically used at 10% or less dilution.
Notes:	Borage seed oil is not recommended for use if pregnant or nursing. If you are currently taking medication, consult with your doctor before use.

Camellia Seed Oil

Price:	$
Shelf life:	Up to 1 year.
Scent:	Herbaceous, with a hint of tea.
Color:	Yellow.
Source:	The seeds of the Camellia flower. This flower grows on tea trees, but this oil is different from tea tree oil, which is an essential oil. Camellia seed oil is sometimes referred to as tea oil.
Good for:	Dry and damaged skin. It heals the skin and protects it from damage without leaving a greasy residue.
Contains:	Oleic acid, linoleic acid, antioxidants, vitamins and minerals.
Dilution:	Typically used at 10% or less dilution.
Notes:	Camellia seed oil is often sold in a diluted version called Camellia oil. For aromatherapy purposes, seek out the undiluted Camellia seed oil.

Castor Oil

Price: $

Shelf life: Up to 1 year.

Scent: None.

Color: Various shades of yellow.

Source: Castor beans.

Good for: Good for all skin types. Leaves protective coating behind that protects skin from the elements.

Contains: Oleic acid and small amounts of linoleic acid.

Dilution: Typically used at 10% or less dilution.

Notes: Castor oil can be used as an emulsifying agent, meaning it helps to disperse other oils into water.

Coconut Oil

Price:	$
Shelf life:	Up to 2 years.
Scent:	Coconut.
Color:	Clear white.
Source:	Coconut pulp.
Good for:	Most skin types, but may irritate sensitive skin. Leaves an oily protective residue.
Contains:	Oleic acid, linoleic acid, vitamins and minerals.
Dilution:	Typically used at 10% to 25% dilution.
Notes:	Coconut oil is solid at room temperature. Heat it just enough to melt it to add it to your oil blends. It can be used to help disperse oils into water.

<u>Evening Primrose Oil</u>

Price:	$$
Shelf life:	Up to 1 year. Keep refrigerated.
Scent:	Sweet.
Color:	Yellow.
Source:	Evening Primrose seeds.
Good for:	All skin types. Used to ease the effects of skin conditions like psoriasis and eczema. Used for problems associated with PMS and menopause. Leaves a slight residue.
Contains:	High linoleic acid content. Also contains oleic acid, vitamins and minerals.
Dilution:	Typically used at 10% or less dilution.
Notes:	Do not heat Evening Primrose oil.

Grapeseed Oil

Price:	$
Shelf life:	Up to 1 year.
Scent:	Light and nutty.
Color:	Almost clear.
Source:	Grape seeds.
Good for:	All skin types. Leaves an oily sheen.
Contains:	High linoleic acid content. Also contains oleic acid, protein, vitamins and minerals.
Dilution:	Used at 100% or as a blend with other carrier oils.
Notes:	Grapeseed oil is an inexpensive all-purpose oil that can be used for most aromatherapy purposes.

Hazelnut Oil

Price:	$
Shelf life:	Up to 1 year.
Scent:	Slightly nutty.
Color:	Pale yellow.
Source:	Hazelnuts.
Good for:	Has astringent qualities. Good for those with oily skin. Leaves a slight residue.
Contains:	High oleic acid content. Also contains linoleic acid, vitamins and minerals.
Dilution:	Typically used at 100%.
Notes:	Hazelnut oil is an inexpensive all-purpose oil that can be used for most aromatherapy purposes, but works best for people with oily skin. Do not use if you have nut allergies.

Hemp Seed Oil

Price:	$ - $$
Shelf life:	Up to 1 year.
Scent:	Slightly nutty.
Color:	Various shades of green.
Source:	The seeds of the hemp plant.
Good for:	All skin types. Considered one of the best oils for cosmetic applications. Leaves a slight sheen behind.
Contains:	Oleic acid, linoleic acid, vitamins and minerals.
Dilution:	Typically used at 100%.
Notes:	Hemp seed oil tends to get a bad rap because of its ties to the cannabis plant. There is no THC in hemp seed oil and it's one of the best carrier oils around.

Jojoba Oil

Price:	$$
Shelf life:	Up to 1 year.
Scent:	Aromatic.
Color:	Yellow.
Source:	Jojoba fruits.
Good for:	All skin types, but best for oily skin. Similar in feel to the sebum emitted by human skin follicles.
Contains:	Oleic acid, protein, vitamins and minerals.
Dilution:	Can be used at higher percentages, but works best when blended at 10% with other carrier oils. Jojoba oil absorbs rapidly into the skin.
Notes:	While it's called an oil, Jojoba oil is technically a liquid wax. Don't let that deter you from using it, as it's a favorite for massage oil blends. Jojoba oil may start to solidify and cloud up at cooler temperatures. Gently warm it to liquefy it.

Macadamia Nut

Price: $

Shelf life: Up to 1 year.

Scent: Strong nutty fragrance.

Color: Clear yellow.

Source: Macadamia nuts.

Good for: All skin types, but best for damaged skin. Lends itself well to massage oil blends. Considered one of the best regenerative oils around.

Contains: High oleic acid content. Doesn't contain a lot of linoleic acid.

Dilution: Use at 10% to 20% dilution for best results.

Notes: Macadamia nut oil can be used to reduce inflammation and regenerate damaged skin. Do not use if you have nut allergies.

Olive Oil

Price: | $

Shelf life: | Up to 2 years.

Scent: | Smells like the olive oil used for cooking purposes. Can influence the fragrance of essential oils, so use with caution.

Color: | Various shades of green.

Source: | Olives.

Good for: | All skin types. Universal oil used for all applications. Leaves behind a slightly oily protective coating.

Contains: | Oleic acid, linoleic acid, vitamins and minerals.

Dilution: | Use at 10% or less dilution for best results.

Notes: | Olive oil is a universal oil that can be used for most purposes. While it can be used for almost anything, that doesn't mean it should, as it's a heavy oil that can overpower a blend if it isn't used with caution.

Pumpkin Seed Oil

Price:	$$
Shelf life:	Up to 1 year.
Scent:	Nutty.
Color:	Dark green.
Source:	Pumpkin seeds.
Good for:	Dry or damaged skin. Leaves a slightly oily protective sheen.
Contains:	Oleic acid, linoleic acid, antioxidants, sterols, vitamins and minerals.
Dilution:	Use at 10% dilution for best results.
Notes:	Pumpkin seed oil is considered one of the healthiest oils on the market today. Do not heat this oil. Do not use if you have nut allergies.

Rosehip Seed Oil

Price: $$ - $$$

Shelf life: Up to 6 months.

Scent: Rich and earthy.

Color: Clear.

Source: Rose seeds.

Good for: All skin types, especially damaged skin. May aggravate acne if used in concentrated amounts. Dries quickly and doesn't leave an oily sheen.

Contains: Oleic acid, linoleic acid, vitamins and minerals.

Dilution: Dilute to 10% or less for best results.

Notes: Rosehip seed oil is great for dry and damaged skin. It can go rancid if it isn't stored properly. Keep in a cool, dark place and refrigerate after opening.

Sesame Seed Oil

Price:	$
Shelf life:	Up to 1 year.
Scent:	Sweet and nutty.
Color:	Yellow.
Source:	Sesame seeds.
Good for:	All skin types. Used to treat skin conditions like eczema and psoriasis. Leaves behind an oily protective coating.
Contains:	Oleic acid, linoleic acid, protein, vitamins and minerals.
Dilution:	Dilute to 10% or less for best results.
Notes:	Sesame seed oil can overpower other oils in a blend if used at higher than the recommended amount.

Sunflower Oil

Price:	$
Shelf life:	Up to 1 year.
Scent:	Sweet and nutty.
Color:	Clear yellow.
Source:	Sunflower seeds.
Good for:	All skin types. Does not leave a residue.
Contains:	Oleic acid, linoleic acid, vitamins and minerals. There is a high-oleic version available that ups the oleic acid content to more than 75%.
Dilution:	Typically used at 100%.
Notes:	Sunflower oil is a good base oil for most aromatherapy oil blends. Do not use if you have nut allergies.

Wheat Germ Oil

Price:	$ - $$
Shelf life:	Up to 1 year.
Scent:	Earthy. Stronger than most carrier oils.
Color:	Yellow to brown.
Source:	Wheat germ.
Good for:	All skin types. Good for dry and damaged skin. Used to treat effects of eczema and psoriasis.
Contains:	Oleic acid, linoleic acid, antioxidants, vitamins and minerals.
Dilution:	Use at 10% or less dilution for best results.
Notes:	Wheat germ oil is sensitive oil that should be refrigerated when not in use. Do not heat wheat germ oil. Do not use if you have wheat allergies.

10 Essential Oils You Should Own

With so many oils on the market to choose from, deciding where to start can lead to analysis paralysis. You want to choose the best oils for you and your family, but you have no clue where to begin.

The 10 oils listed in this section are a good start. These oils will give you a wide range of therapeutic benefits and won't break the bank, even if you buy all 10 at once. Once you own these oils, you can mix and match the rest of the oils listed in the next section to better suit your personal needs. If you don't currently have these essential oils in your collection, you should. Buy them one at a time as you can afford them or all at once. Just make sure you have them ready when you need them.

#1: Lavender

Lavender oil is probably the best known and most popular essential oil on the market today. It's calming and aromatic and has a wide array of healing properties. From helping promote the healing of wounds and burns to relieving aches and pains, lavender essential oil has you covered. One minor warning before you take out stock in lavender oil, the scent of lavender oil is somewhat of an acquired taste that some people don't care for at first. Once you get used to it, you'll learn to love it.

Lavender Oil Information

Price:	$ - $$
Scent:	Green, floral and sweet.
Note:	Thin top to middle notes.
Color:	Yellow.
Source:	Lavender flowers.
Properties:	Analgesic, anticonvulsant, antidepressant, antiseptic, antispasmodic, antiviral, calming, deodorant, relaxing.
Good for:	Acne, aches and pains, cuts and burns, deodorant, scars and stretch marks, insect bites, itching, respiratory conditions, skin conditions, stress relief.
Contains:	Linalol, linalyl acetate and more.
Strength:	Mild.
Blends well with:	Most oils.

Safety concerns: None that I'm aware of.

#2: Roman Chamomile

Roman chamomile essential oil is great for those days when you're feeling down in the dumps or stressed out because its calming and relaxing properties can soothe the soul. It can help soothe frayed nerves and is one of the few oils generally considered safe for use with children in small amounts. Ladies, it's also good to have around for that time of the month. It can help ease some of the stress and pain associated with PMS.

Roman Chamomile Oil Information

Price:	$$
Scent:	Green, floral and sweet.
Note:	Strong middle notes.
Color:	Clear with a blue tint.
Source:	Chamomile flowers.
Properties:	Analgesic, antibacterial, antibiotic, antidepressant, anti-inflammatory, antimicrobial, antiseptic, antispasmodic, calming, sedative, skin healing, tonic.
Good for:	Aches and pains, arthritis, cuts and burns, depression, hair care, insect bites, mood disorders, PMS, PTSD, sedative, skin disorders, stress relief, toothache.
Contains:	Azulene, bisabolol, camphene, esters, pinocarvene, pinene and more.
Strength:	Medium. May cause skin irritation. Dilute for best results.
Blends well	Citrus oils, clary sage, floral oils,

with: frankincense, lavender, patchouli, ylang ylang.

Safety concerns: Non-toxic. Avoid during pregnancy. Those with allergies to ragweed should avoid use of this oil.

#3: Eucalyptus

If you've ever spent time in a grove of Eucalyptus trees, you've enjoyed the scent of eucalyptus oil. This oil has a number of therapeutic uses, but it's most widely used for easing congestion and coughs. It also has a cooling effect on the skin and can be used to treat inflammation and skin conditions. This versatile oil is one everybody should have in their medicine cabinet.

Eucalyptus Oil Information

Price:	$ - $$
Scent:	Fresh and distinct. Smells like eucalyptus trees.
Note:	Strong top notes.
Color:	Clear.
Source:	Leaves and twigs of eucalyptus trees.
Properties:	Analgesic, antibacterial, anti-inflammatory, antimicrobial, antiseptic, antispasmodic, cooling, decongestant, expectorant, deodorant, immune system stimulant.
Good for:	Aches and pains, arthritis, coughing, fevers, headaches, improved circulation, skin care.
Contains:	α-pinene , b-pinene, camphene, cineole, limonene, pinocarvene and more.
Strength:	Medium. May cause skin irritation. Dilute heavily for best results.
Blends well	Citrus oils, clary sage, lavender, jasmine, patchouli, peppermint, tea tree,

with: ylang ylang.

Safety concerns: Toxic when ingested orally. Avoid
                     while pregnant.

#4: Lemon

You're going to want to have at least one type of citrus oil on hand to start. I chose lemon essential oil because of its invigorating and refreshing scent that's capable of making short work of even the most stubborn of odors. Lemon oil blends well with a number of popular oils and has a lot of therapeutic uses.

I went with lemon oil as my top ten citrus oil because I love the scent. You could pick orange, lime or grapefruit and get pretty much the same effect. Your call.

Lemon Oil Information

Price:	$
Scent:	Smells like lemon.
Note:	Strong top notes.
Color:	Yellow.
Source:	Lemon peels.
Properties:	Antibacterial, antifungal, anti-inflammatory, antimicrobial, antiseptic, antispasmodic, astringent, carminative, cleansing, digestive, diuretic, deodorant, refreshing, stimulant.
Good for:	Cold relief, detox, fever relief, fatigue, improves circulation, insect bites, oily skin, wounds, wrinkles.
Contains:	α-pinene , b-pinene, citral, geranial, limonene and more.
Strength:	Medium. May cause skin irritation. Dilute heavily before use.

Blends well with:	Chamomile, citrus oils, eucalyptus, frankincense, geranium, lavender, rose, sandalwood, ylang ylang.
Safety concerns:	Can cause skin irritation, especially if used undiluted. Phototoxic.

#5: Frankincense

Frankincense essential oil is a wood resin-derived oil that's been around since Biblical times. It's one of the oils that the wise men brought to baby Jesus in the Bible. In addition to uplifting spiritual applications, this aromatic oil is good for relief from respiratory problems and skin conditions.

Frankincense Oil Information

Price:	$$ - $$$
Scent:	Woody and campherous.
Note:	Base.
Color:	Clear yellow.
Source:	Frankincense tree resin.
Properties:	Analgesic, antibacterial, antifungal, anti-inflammatory, antiseptic, astringent, carminative, digestive, diuretic, sedative, tonic.
Good for:	Acid reflux, anxiety, cold and flu relief, damaged skin, dry skin, scars, skin care, stress, wrinkles.
Contains:	Borneol, limonene, pinene, farnesol and more.
Strength:	Mild.
Blends well with:	Benzoin, citrus oils, lavender, myrrh, pine.
Safety concerns:	None that I'm aware of.

#6: Tea Tree

Tea tree essential oil is one of the few oils I can't live without. It's not the best-smelling oil around, but it has so many health benefits that you'll learn to love its herbaceous scent. You're going to want to have this oil on hand for those times when you have to clean out a wound or aren't feeling well. It can be used to ease the effects of a number of viral and fungal infections while boosting the immune system in the process.

Tea Tree Oil Information

Price:	$ - $$
Scent:	Herbaceous.
Note:	Middle.
Color:	Clear yellow.
Source:	Leaves and twigs from the tea tree.
Properties:	Analgesic, antibacterial, antifungal, anti-inflammatory, antimicrobial, antiparasitic, antiseptic, antiviral, decongestant, deodorant, expectorant, insect repellent, stimulant.
Good for:	Acne, burns, cold and flu relief, dandruff, fever, fungal outbreaks, immune system, infections, insect bites, respiratory conditions, sunburn, wounds.
Contains:	Cineol, pinene, terpenene, terpineol and more.
Strength:	Mild to medium. Can cause skin irritation. Dilute before use.

Blends well with:	Basil, chamomile, cinnamon, clary sage, lavender, spice oils, ylang ylang.
Safety concerns:	Can cause sensitization issues. Avoid using at full strength.

#7: Ylang Ylang

Ylang ylang oil is one of the best oils for relieving depression, stress and other emotional conditions. It soothes the nerves and calms the soul. It balances the skin at the same time. Oh yeah, it smells great and is an aphrodisiac to boot. What more could you ask for in an oil?

There are multiple varieties of ylang ylang oil available based on when the oil is removed from the distillation process. Ylang ylang "extra" is extracted at the beginning of the process and is considered the best for aromatherapy purposes. It's also the most expensive. Grades I, II and III are progressively less expensive, but don't have the same quality as the "extra" grade oil.

Don't let the price of "extra" deter you. The other grades can be used if you don't want to spend the money for the more expensive oil.

Ylang Ylang Oil Information

Price:	$$ - $$$
Scent:	Sweet, floral and heady.
Note:	Middle.
Color:	Clear yellow.
Source:	Ylang ylang flowers.
Properties:	Antibacterial, antidepressant, antifungal, anti-inflammatory, antiseptic, antispasmodic, aphrodisiac, disinfectant, expectorant, sedative.
Good for:	Anger management, cold and flu, emotional issues, headache, insomnia,

scars, stress relief, wounds.

Contains:	Various constituents based on the distillation. It could contain acetates, ethers, eugenol, farnesol, linalol, geraniol and pinene, amongst other compounds.
Strength:	Medium. Dilute heavily before use.
Blends well with:	Chamomile, citrus oils, clary sage, lavender, sandalwood.
Safety concerns:	Can cause upset stomach and headaches when too much of this oil is used. Possible skin irritant, so always dilute.

#8: Peppermint

Peppermint essential oil is another all-purpose oil that you're going to want on hand. It's an all-natural bug repellant that will drive pesky insects from your home without use of poisonous chemicals. It has cooling properties and works well to ease the effects of nausea and headaches. It's also one of the strongest expectorant oils you can buy.

Peppermint Oil Information

Price:	$$ - $$$
Scent:	Minty, fresh.
Note:	Intense top note.
Color:	Clear yellow.
Source:	Peppermint leaves.
Properties:	Analgesic, antibacterial, anti-inflammatory, antifungal, antimicrobial, antiseptic, antispasmodic, astringent, expectorant, insect repellent, sedative, stimulant.
Good for:	Aches and pains, clarity of mind, fatigue, focus, nausea, respiratory disorders, skin care, skin irritation, skin inflammation, sunburn, vertigo.
Contains:	Cineole, limonene, menthol, menthone, pinene, pulegone and more.
Strength:	Strong. Dilute heavily before use.
Blends well with:	Campherous oils, citrus oils, eucalyptus, lavender, rosemary.

Safety concerns: Pregnant women and those prone to
seizures should avoid this oil. It can be a
skin irritant, so dilute heavily before use.

#9: Rosemary

Rosemary essential oil is like the Swiss Army knife of essential oils. It does a little bit of everything. It's a strong stimulant that will leave you feeling invigorated and alive. It works great when you're feeling under the weather and want relief from a cough or cold and it's good for your skin. You can even use this oil to help ease the effects of a hangover.

There are two common types of rosemary oil. Rosemary cineole is the stronger of the two and contains more camphor than the other type, making it ideal for treating respiratory conditions like asthma and coughing. Rosemary verbenone is the milder version and is the preferred choice for topical application because it isn't as harsh.

Rosemary Oil Information

Price:	$ - $$
Scent:	Herbaceous, medicinal.
Note:	Strong middle to base.
Color:	Clear yellow.
Source:	Rosemary herb.
Properties:	Analgesic, antibacterial, antifungal, antioxidant, antiseptic, antispasmodic, aphrodisiac, astringent, carminative, decongestant, disinfectant, diuretic, expectorant, stimulant, tonic.
Good for:	Aches and pains, arthritis, circulation, cold and flu, coughs, dandruff, hair care, hangover, insect repellent, memory,

sinus disorders, wounds.

Contains:	Camphene, camphor, cineole, ketones, limonene, linalol, oxides, pinene, thujone and more.
Strength:	Mild.
Blends well with:	Citrus oils, Cedarwood, spice oils.
Safety concerns:	Do not use when pregnant or if you're prone to seizures.

#10: Vetiver

Looking to unwind after a long, hard day? If so, Vetiver essential oil has you covered. I've found Vetiver is one of the most relaxing and soothing oils there is. In addition to promoting emotional well-being, Vetiver also soothes and eases the effects of numerous skin conditions. Be careful when using this powerful oil. A little Vetiver goes a long way.

Vetiver Oil Information

Price:	$ - $$
Scent:	Deep and earthy.
Note:	Powerful base note.
Color:	Brown.
Source:	Vetiver grass.
Properties:	Analgesic, antibacterial, antifungal, anti-inflammatory, antioxidant, antiseptic, sedative, stimulant, tonic.
Good for:	Aches and pains, anxiety, cuts and burns, fades scars, insect bites, insomnia, PMS, skin care, stress relief, tension.
Contains:	Benzoic acid, vetiverol, furfurol and more.
Strength:	Weak. Needs to be heavily diluted to avoid overpowering scent. Dilute to less than 2%.
Blends well with:	Most other oils.

Safety concerns: None that I'm aware of.

Additional Oils You Might Want to Own

There's one thing about essential oils that I probably should have warned you about sooner. Once you start buying and using them and reaping their benefits, it can get a bit addictive. The ten oils in the previous chapter are a great start, but you're soon going to find you want to expand on that list in order to create super blends that maximize certain therapeutic qualities.

Another good reason to expand outward is to try to find the oils that best suit your personal needs. While I tried to pick oils that are beneficial to most people in the previous chapter, you may find your body doesn't react positively to certain oils. If that happens, don't worry. It's natural. Everyone's body is different and we all have different chemical balances. Discontinue use of the oil that doesn't agree with you and seek out oils with similar properties that do agree with your body. Aromatherapy isn't a one size fits all type deal. I'm of the belief that there's a good fit for everyone, it's just not one size fits all. What works well for one person may not work at all for another. It's up to you to determine what does and doesn't work. There are hundreds of oils out there, so don't give up right away if an oil you buy isn't a good fit. Keep searching and try to find something is.

The rest of the chapter is packed full of popular oils that may have qualities you're interested in. Add oils that fill your needs to your collection as you can afford them. Soon you'll have a collection with all sorts of therapeutic benefits.

NOTE: The information in this section is not complete, nor is it the final word on essential oils. The world of essential oils is a complex one and we're just now beginning to understand just how powerful they are. Proceed with caution and always consult with your physician prior to using essential oils. This is especially important if you have health issues that the oils may aggravate.

Allspice

Allspice essential oil isn't a front-runner on most people's list of favorite oils. That said, it does have its uses. It has warming qualities and penetrates deep into the skin to ease muscle and rheumatism pains. It works well in oil blends designed to alleviate aches and pains. It's also used to relieve stress and ease tension.

Allspice Oil Information

Price:	$$ - $$$
Scent:	Strong cinnamon and clove fragrance.
Note:	Heavy middle.
Color:	Brown.
Source:	Pimenta berries.
Properties:	Analgesic, anesthetic, antibacterial, antifungal, antioxidant, antiseptic, antiviral, aphrodisiac.
Good for:	Aches and pains, arthritis, cold relief, muscle cramping, nausea, respiratory conditions, stress relief.
Contains:	Cineol, eugenol and more.
Strength:	Strong. Dilute heavily before use.
Blends well with:	Citrus oils, spice oils.
Safety concerns:	Can irritate skin and mucous membranes. Must be diluted heavily before use. Do not use if pregnant.

Angelica Root

Angelica root essential oil is expensive, but has a number of great qualities. My favorite is that it helps ease cramping and other symptoms associated with PMS. It's also said to help with problems associated with menopause. It boosts the immune system and helps ward off infections and viruses.

Angelica Root Oil Information

Price:	$$$ - $$$$
Scent:	Peppery and spicy.
Note:	Base.
Color:	Clear yellow.
Source:	Angelica root.
Properties:	Antibacterial, antifungal, antispasmodic, carminative, digestive, diuretic, expectorant, stimulant, tonic.
Good for:	Anemia, arthritis, colds, menopause, PMS, respiratory conditions, removal of toxins, skin care, stress relief.
Contains:	Bisabolene, camphene, limonene, pinene and more.
Strength:	Mild.
Blends well with:	Cedarwood, citrus oils, myrrh, patchouli.
Safety concerns:	Avoid while pregnant. Avoid if you have diabetes. Phototoxic. May attract insects.

Anise

Anise essential oil is interesting in that it has the strong scent of black licorice. Hunters and fishermen use the scent of anise to mask their human scent to make them undetectable to their prey. Anise oil can also be used to help ease the effects of colds and the flu. Nursing women can use it to stimulate the production of breast milk.

Anise Oil Information

Price:	$
Scent:	Black licorice.
Note:	Top to middle.
Color:	Clear.
Source:	Anise plant.
Properties:	Analgesic, antiseptic, antispasmodic, calming, carminative, digestive, diuretic, expectorant, stimulant.
Good for:	Colds, insect bites, stimulates breast milk production, stress relief, respiratory conditions.
Contains:	Camphene, linalool, pinene, safrole and more.
Strength:	Strong. Dilute heavily before use.
Blends well with:	Wood oils.
Safety concerns:	Those with sensitive or damaged skin should avoid this oil as it can cause sensitization issues. Do not use if you have poor circulation, as it may slow circulation further. Avoid aniseed oil

while pregnant because it contains a chemical that can start menstruation.

Basil

Basil essential oil is a great choice for those days where you know you're going to be on the run all day. Use it in the morning and you might find you're able to focus and still get stuff done well after you normally would have worn down. Basil oil contains methyl chavicol, which is a possible carcinogen, so avoid relying too heavily on this oil. Use it infrequently and in small amounts when you need an emotional boost.

Basil Oil Information

Price:	$ - $$
Scent:	Spicy and fresh.
Note:	Strong top.
Color:	Yellow to brown.
Source:	Basil leaves.
Properties:	Antibacterial, antidepressant, antiseptic, antispasmodic, carminative, expectorant, stimulant, tonic.
Good for:	Allergies, cuts and burns, cold and flu, fatigue, focus, insect bites, insect repellent, motivation, respiratory conditions, stress relief.
Contains:	Camphene, eugenol, limonene, linalool, methyl chavicol, methyl cinnamate and more.
Strength:	Strong. Dilute heavily, as large doses may be carcinogenic.

Blends well with: Citrus oils, lavender, neroli.

Safety concerns: Do not use if pregnant or if you have other health conditions. Contains methyl chavicol, which may be carcinogenic.

Bay Laurel

Bay Laurel essential oil is a great choice for when you need a little confidence boost. It also works well as an expectorant for those days when you're feeling all clogged up and want some relief. Be aware that bay laurel oil and bay oil are two different beasts. Bay oil has warming properties (amongst other things) that bay laurel oil doesn't have.

Bay Laurel Oil Information

Price:	$$
Scent:	Campherous and clean.
Note:	Top to middle.
Color:	Yellow.
Source:	Bay laurel leaves.
Properties:	Analgesic, anesthetic, antifungal, antimicrobial, antiseptic, carminative, sedative.
Good for:	Aches and pains, cold and flu, confidence, infection, insomnia, mental stability.
Contains:	Pinene, limonene, linalool, methyl chavicol, myrcene and more.
Strength:	Strong. Dilute heavily, as large doses may be carcinogenic. This oil can cause skin irritation and sensitization issues.
Blends well with:	Spice oils.
Safety concerns:	Do not use if pregnant or if you have

other health conditions. Contains
methyl chavicol, which may be
carcinogenic.

Bergamot

Bergamot essential oil is a refreshing citrus oil that smells sweet with a bit of spice added in for good measure. Unless you're familiar with essential oils, you probably haven't heard of the bergamot fruit because it's inedible. Bergamot oil's astringent qualities make it a good choice for those with oily skin. It stimulates the mind and can be used when you're looking for a pick-me-up when feeling sad or blue. Bergamot oil is more expensive than the more common oils like lemon, lime and grapefruit, but it's worth putting out the extra money for the interesting fragrance and its therapeutic qualities.

This oil is a good choice for crafting a natural deodorant to replace the synthetic deodorants most people use. Mix a drop or two of bergamot and a drop or two of lavender oil into a carrier oil and apply. It'll leave you smelling clean and fresh all day long.

Bergamot Oil Information

Price:	$$
Scent:	Spicy citrus.
Note:	Top.
Color:	Green.
Source:	Bergamot peels.
Properties:	Analgesic, antidepressant, antiseptic, antibiotic, antispasmodic, astringent, calming, deodorant.
Good for:	Cleansing, depression, fatigue, infection, oily skin, respiratory

conditions, skin care, stress relief.

Contains:	Bergaptene, bisabolene, limonene, linalool, myrcene, nerol, pinene, terpenol and more.
Strength:	Medium. Dilute heavily before use.
Blends well with:	Citrus oils, floral oils, spice oils.
Safety concerns:	Phototoxic. Seek out bergaptene-free versions of bergamot oil to lessen or eliminate the phototoxicity.

Black Pepper

Black pepper oil has an amazing scent that adds a bit of spice to your oil blends. The warming qualities of this oil make it a good choice for relieving muscle aches and pains and it's said to improve circulation.

Black Pepper Oil Information

Price:	$$ - $$$
Scent:	Spicy and peppery.
Note:	Middle.
Color:	Green to light brown.
Source:	Peppercorns.
Properties:	Analgesic, antiseptic, antispasmodic, aphrodisiac, carminative, tonic, warming.
Good for:	Circulation, cold and flu, fatigue, hangover relief, muscle aches and pains.
Contains:	Bisabolene, camphene, limonene, linalool, pinene, terpenene, thujone and more.
Strength:	Medium. Dilute heavily for best results.
Blends well with:	Floral oils, spice oils.
Safety concerns:	Possible skin irritant. Avoid while pregnant.

Cajuput

Cajuput, or cajeput as it's called in some literature, essential oil is one of my personal favorite oils. I debated including it as one of the oils in the Top Ten list in the previous chapter, but it was barely edged out by Vetiver oil. Use it when you feel a cold coming on to help ward it off. This is anecdotal at best, but I feel that my colds and illnesses aren't anywhere near as bad when I use cajuput oil as soon as I feel one coming on. Cajuput oil is inexpensive, so it should be one of the first oils you add to your collection after you get the Top Ten.

Cajuput Oil Information

Price:	$
Scent:	Campherous, slight medicinal.
Note:	Middle.
Color:	Clear yellow.
Source:	Cajuput leaves and twigs.
Properties:	Analgesic, antifungal, antimicrobial, antiseptic, antispasmodic, expectorant, insect repellent.
Good for:	Aches and pains, circulation, cold and flu, fatigue, insect bites and stings,
Contains:	Cineole, linalool, myrcene, pinene, terpenene and more.
Strength:	Medium. Dilute heavily before use.
Blends well with:	Spice oils.
Safety concerns:	Possible dermal irritant.

Chamomile, German

There are two basic types of chamomile oil. We discussed Roman chamomile oil in the previous chapter. While the scents of the two oils are somewhat similar and both have calming properties, there are some key differences. Roman chamomile is more effective when used for mood-altering applications, while German chamomile is best used to treat skin conditions. German chamomile contains azulene, which makes it a good choice to reduce inflammation.

German Chamomile Oil Information

Price:	$$$
Scent:	Floral and sweet.
Note:	Middle.
Color:	Blue.
Source:	Matricaria chamomilla plant.
Properties:	Analgesic, antibiotic, anti-inflammatory, antispasmodic, carminative, sedative.
Good for:	Calming, inflammation, menopause, PMS, skin conditions, skin care, stress relief.
Contains:	Azulene, bisabolol, farnasene, farnesol and more.
Strength:	Mild to medium. Dilute heavily before use for best results.
Blends well with:	Citrus oils, clary sage, lavender, rose, ylang ylang.
Safety concerns:	Do not use while pregnant.

Cedarwood

Cedarwood essential oil is a spiritual oil enjoyed by those who use aromatherapy to uplift their spirits and improve their moods. It also sees use for skin care applications and is passable as an expectorant.

Be sure to obtain your Cedarwood oil from sustainably harvested sources. Cedar trees can live for thousands of years, but old-growth trees in some areas are relatively rare because of overharvest. Cedarwood oils from locations in the United States are your best bet for sustainably harvested oils.

Cedarwood Oil Information

Price:	$
Scent:	Woody. Smells like cedar.
Note:	Base.
Color:	Golden yellow.
Source:	Cedar wood.
Properties:	Antiseptic, antispasmodic, astringent, expectorant, insect repellent, sedative.
Good for:	Acne, arthritis, cold relief, itching, mood enhancement, oily skin, respiratory conditions, stress relief, tension.
Contains:	Cedrene, cedrol, thujopsene, widdrol and more.
Strength:	Medium. Dilute well for best results.
Blends well with:	Citrus oils,

Safety concerns: May cause dermal or mucous membrane irritation. Do not use if pregnant.

Cinnamon Bark

There are a number of variations of cinnamon oil on the market today. If you want the smell of cinnamon, go with cinnamon bark essential oil over cinnamon leaf oil, which has a scent closer to that of cloves. Be aware that this oil is extremely powerful and is a strong dermal and mucous membrane irritant. It should only be used in tiny amounts.

Cinnamon Bark Oil Information

Price:	$ - $$$
Scent:	Cinnamon.
Note:	Strong middle.
Color:	Brown.
Source:	The bark of the cinnamon tree.
Properties:	Analgesic, antibacterial, antifungal, anti-inflammatory, antimicrobial, antiseptic, antispasmodic, aphrodisiac, astringent, carminative, expectorant.
Good for:	Air freshener, circulation, disinfectant, cold relief, fatigue, insect bites, stress relief.
Contains:	Cinnamaldehyde, eugenol and more.
Strength:	Very strong. Do not apply topically.
Blends well with:	Most essential oils.
Safety concerns:	Strong dermal and mucous membrane irritant. Do not use while pregnant. Do not apply topically. Phototoxic. Use only with the approval of your

doctor and under the supervision of an aromatherapy practitioner.

Citronella

Those who live in an area where insect infestations are a problem are going to want to have citronella essential oil on hand. It works well to get rid of most pesky bugs, including fleas, mosquitos and bees. The most common use for citronella is to add it to candles that are used in the backyard or on camping trips to keep insects at bay. A few strategically-placed candles can work wonders when the bugs get too thick to handle. It's also capable of altering your mood and can be used to clear your mind so you can better focus on the task at hand

<u>Citronella Oil Information</u>

Price:	$
Scent:	Lemony, clean and refreshing.
Note:	Top.
Color:	Clear.
Source:	Citronella grass.
Properties:	Analgesic, antibacterial, antifungal, antiseptic, antispasmodic, astringent, deodorant, insect repellent, stimulant, tonic.
Good for:	Clearing the mind, focus, insect repellent, skin care.
Contains:	Borneol, camphene, citronellol, geraniol and more.
Strength:	Strong. Probably best to avoid contact with skin.
Blends well with:	Citrus oils, lavender.

Safety concerns: Do not use when pregnant. Possible
                     dermal irritant.

Clary Sage

Clary sage oil has a uniquely grassy and slightly bitter aroma that adds an interesting fragrance to oil blends when used in moderation. It's thought to create harmonious mental balance and has seen use to ease the effects of PMS and menopause.

Clary Sage Oil Information

Price:	$$ - $$$
Scent:	Grassy, earthy and herbaceous.
Note:	Middle.
Color:	Yellow.
Source:	Clary sage leaves and flowers.
Properties:	Antibacterial, antifungal, anti-inflammatory, antispasmodic, aphrodisiac, tonic, sedative, relaxant, deodorant, carminative,
Good for:	Aches and pains, balance, cramping, dandruff, fatigue, harmony, stress relief, skin conditions.
Contains:	Linalool, linalyl acetate, myrcene, pinene and more.
Strength:	Mild. Dilute before topical application.
Blends well with:	Most essential oils.
Safety concerns:	Do not use when pregnant.

Dill

Dill essential oil works well on two fronts. It helps heal damaged skin and may reduce scarring. People who are stressed out or prone to panic attacks can use it to help calm their nerves.

Dill Oil Information

Price:	$ - $$
Scent:	Grassy, sweet and earthy.
Note:	Top to middle.
Color:	Clear.
Source:	Dill herb or seeds.
Properties:	Antibacterial, antispasmodic, carminative, insect repellent, stimulant.
Good for:	Cramping, fatigue, flatulence, headaches, insect repellent, panic, overwhelmed feelings, sadness, well-being.
Contains:	Carvone, dillapiol, eugenol, limonene, terpenene and more.
Strength:	Mild.
Blends well with:	Citrus oils.
Safety concerns:	None that I'm aware of.

Fennel Seed

Do you have a big presentation coming up at work or something you're feeling nervous or anxious about? Using fennel essential oil an hour or so before the presentation may enable you to build up the courage to knock it out of the park. Fennel seed oil is also thought to fight obesity and is good for most skin types. Make sure you get sweet fennel oil, as the bitter variety shouldn't be used for aromatherapy.

Fennel Oil Information

Price:	$$
Scent:	Sweet and aromatic. Similar to black licorice.
Note:	Top.
Color:	Yellow.
Source:	Fennel seeds.
Properties:	Analgesic, antibacterial, antifungal, anti-inflammatory, antimicrobial, antispasmodic, expectorant, narcotic, stimulant, tonic.
Good for:	Bruises, courage, cramps, hangover relief, oily skin, strength.
Contains:	Anethole, fenchone, limonene, pinene, thymol and more.
Strength:	Strong. Dilute heavily before use for best results.
Blends well with:	Black pepper, citrus oils, dill, lavender, pine, sandalwood.
Safety concerns:	Possible skin irritant. Avoid while

pregnant or if epileptic. There is some literature that says this oil promotes breast milk production. While that may be true, it contains anethole, which shouldn't be used while nursing.

Geranium

Geranium essential oil works well for skin care purposes. Its floral scent is uplifting and can help ease the mind when you're feeling stressed out.

Geranium Oil Information

Price:	$$ - $$$
Scent:	Floral.
Note:	Strong middle.
Color:	Yellow to brown.
Source:	Geranium leaves.
Properties:	Astringent, calming, deodorant, soothing, tonic.
Good for:	Acne, bruising, skin conditions, PMS, stress relief.
Contains:	Acetates, citronellol, geraniol and more.
Strength:	Medium. Dilute heavily before use.
Blends well with:	Floral oils.
Safety concerns:	May cause dermatitis. Avoid use during pregnancy.

Geranium, Rose

Rose geranium essential oil has been around for a long time. It's seen use as a cure-all for both physical wounds and emotional distress. The best part is it works well for almost all skin types.

Rose Geranium Oil Information

Price:	$$ - $$$
Scent:	Floral.
Note:	Middle.
Color:	Yellow.
Source:	Geranium leaves.
Properties:	Analgesic, antibacterial, anti-inflammatory, antiseptic, astringent, deodorant, insect repellent, sedative, tonic, uplifting.
Good for:	Anxiety, bruises, cuts and burns, damaged skin, insect bites, insect repellent, skin care, skin conditions, stress relief.
Contains:	Citronellol, geraniol, linalool, menthone, pinene and more.
Strength:	Medium. Can cause irritation for some people. Dilute before use.
Blends well with:	Basil, citrus oils, citronella, clary sage, jasmine, lavender, rosemary.
Safety concerns:	Do not use if pregnant.

Ginger

I debated whether or not to include ginger oil in this book, as it's a powerful oil that should only be used under the supervision of a professional, but decided to include it because of its many therapeutic benefits (listed below). Be very careful when using this oil, as it can cause problems if it isn't heavily diluted before use.

Ginger Oil Information

Price:	$$
Scent:	Spicy. Smells like ginger, only stronger.
Note:	Strong base.
Color:	Yellow.
Source:	Ginger root.
Properties:	Analgesic, antibacterial, anticoagulant, anti-inflammatory, antioxidant, antispasmodic, aphrodisiac, astringent, expectorant, stimulant, tonic.
Good for:	Aches and pains, bruising, circulation, colds, cramping, hangover relief, headaches, motion sickness, nausea, respiratory conditions,
Contains:	Borneol, camphene, cineole, linalool, pinene and more.
Strength:	Strong. Dilute heavily before use.
Blends well with:	Citrus and spice oils.

Safety concerns: Strong dermal irritant. Phototoxic.

Grapefruit

Grapefruit essential oil has a sweet citrus scent to it that's refreshing and cleansing. If you're expecting a scent with a bitter edge to it similar to grapefruit, you're going to be pleasantly surprised. White and pink grapefruit oils are both available, with the white being a tad bit sharper than the pink. I'm a big fan of the pink, but the white will work if that's all you can find.

Grapefruit Oil Information

Price:	$ - $$
Scent:	Sweet grapefruit.
Note:	Top.
Color:	Yellow.
Source:	Grapefruit peels.
Properties:	Antibacterial, antidepressant, antioxidant, antiseptic, astringent, cleansing, restorative, stimulant, tonic.
Good for:	Circulation, cold and flu, fatigue, hangover relief, oily skin, stress, stretch marks.
Contains:	Limonene, geraniol, citral and more.
Strength:	Mild, but can irritate the skin. Dilute before use.
Blends well with:	Basil, citrus oils, frankincense, peppermint, wood oils.
Safety concerns:	Phototoxic.

Hyssop

Quality hyssop essential oil demands a premium price, but it's a good oil to have on hand when that time of the month rolls around. It's thought to help with PMS and to ease water retention. It also has expectorant qualities and can be used in blends designed to ease respiratory issues.

Hyssop Oil Information

Price:	$$ - $$$
Scent:	Earthy and sweet.
Note:	Middle.
Color:	Clear to pale green.
Source:	Hyssop plant leaves and flowers.
Properties:	Antibacterial, antiseptic, antispasmodic, antiviral, astringent, expectorant, sedative, tonic.
Good for:	Cuts and scrapes, PMS, respiratory conditions, water retention.
Contains:	Camphene, limonene, pinene, pinocamphene, thujone and more.
Strength:	Mild to medium. Dilute heavily before use.
Blends well with:	Clary sage, orange, melissa.
Safety concerns:	Possibly toxic and neurotoxic. Do not ingest. Do not use if pregnant or epileptic.

Jasmine

Jasmine is a highly sought-after and exquisite oil with an exotic floral aroma. Between a thousand and two thousand pounds of jasmine blossoms are consumed for every pound of jasmine oil that's created. In addition to smelling great, jasmine essential oil has aphrodisiac and mood-enhancing qualities. If you can afford it, it's a great addition to any essential oil collection.

Jasmine Oil Information

Price:	$$$$
Scent:	Intricately floral.
Note:	Middle.
Color:	Amber.
Source:	Jasmine blossoms.
Properties:	Antidepressant, antiseptic, aphrodisiac, expectorant, relaxing, sedative.
Good for:	Breast milk production, depression, dry and irritated skin, impotence, nervousness, respiratory conditions, stress relief.
Contains:	Benzyl acetate and alcohol, geraniol, indole, linalool and more.
Strength:	Mild.
Blends well with:	Citrus oils.
Safety concerns:	May cause an allergic reaction.

Lavandin

While it comes from a plant that's related to lavender oil, lavandin essential oil is a different beast. It doesn't have the same therapeutic qualities as lavender, but is a decent oil in its own right. It can be used to ease respiratory conditions and aches and pains.

Lavandin Oil Information

Price:	$
Scent:	Like lavender, but harsher.
Note:	Top.
Color:	Pale yellow.
Source:	Lavandin flowers.
Properties:	Analgesic, antidepressant, antiseptic, expectorant.
Good for:	Aches and pains, cuts and burns, respiratory conditions.
Contains:	Linalool, linalyl acetate, camphor, cineole and more.
Strength:	Mild. Dilute heavily before use because of its camphor content.
Blends well with:	Bergamot, camphor, citronella, lavender, pine, patchouli, spice oils.
Safety concerns:	Contains camphor. Avoid use while pregnant or if suffering from epilepsy.

Lemongrass

Lemongrass essential oil has been around for hundreds of years. It's one of the few non-citrus oils that contain limonene. It smells like citrus, but is derived from a grass. It has cleansing and deodorant properties and works well in massage oil blends because it helps ease tension and aches and pains. The insect repellent qualities of lemongrass oil make it a passable replacement for citronella if you aren't a big fan of its scent.

Lemongrass Oil Information

Price:	$$
Scent:	Lemon.
Note:	Top.
Color:	Yellow.
Source:	Lemongrass.
Properties:	Analgesic, antidepressant, antifungal, antimicrobial, antiseptic, astringent, cleansing, deodorant, insect repellent, tonic.
Good for:	Acne aches and pains, bruising, fatigue, headaches, insect repellent, nervous system, skin care, stress relief.
Contains:	Citronellol, geraniol, limonene, myrcene, nerol and more.
Strength:	Medium. Possible skin irritant, so dilute heavily.
Blends well with:	Coriander, jasmine, lavender, spice

oils, tea tree.

Safety concerns: May be a dermal irritant.

Melissa

Melissa, or lemon balm, essential oil is great to have on hand if you can afford it. It's one of the most expensive oils on the market today because it takes as much as 7 tons of Melissa plants to make a single pound of oil. It's worth the money because it's one of the stronger medicinal oils available. Beware of companies selling Melissa oil for bargain basement prices. It's usually adulterated with citronella oil and lemongrass, which creates a similar but nowhere near as effective blend.

Melissa Oil Information

Price:	$$$ - $$$$
Scent:	Fresh citrus.
Note:	Middle
Color:	Yellow.
Source:	Lemon balm leaves.
Properties:	Antibacterial, anti-inflammatory, antiseptic, antispasmodic, antiviral, calming, insect repellent, nervine, sedative, tonic.
Good for:	Anxiety, blood pressure, cold and flu, fever, headache, insomnia, insect bites, insect repellent, nausea, PMS, stress relief, tonic.
Contains:	Aesculetine, citronellal, geranial, neral and more.
Strength:	Medium. Dilute heavily for best results.

Blends well with: Roman chamomile, rose, frankincense, spice oils.

Safety concerns: Can be dermal irritant if not diluted appropriately.

Myrrh

You've probably heard of myrrh. Along with frankincense, myrrh was one of the oils the wise men brought to Jesus in the Bible. Myrrh oil has a pleasant fragrance and is a great oil to use when you want emotional stability and well-being.

Myrrh Oil Information

Price:	$$ - $$$
Scent:	Deep balsamic.
Note:	Base.
Color:	Amber.
Source:	Resin from the myrrh tree.
Properties:	Anticatarrhal, antifungal, anti-inflammatory, antimicrobial, antiseptic, antiviral, astringent, carminative, expectorant, sedative, tonic.
Good for:	Athlete's foot, calming, relaxing, old and flu, damaged skin, skin care, respiratory conditions, wrinkles.
Contains:	Acetic acid, cadinene, eugenol, formic acid, limonene, pinene and more.
Strength:	Mild to medium. Dilute heavily for best results.
Blends well with:	Citrus oils, frankincense, lavender, sandalwood, tea tree, ylang ylang.
Safety concerns:	Toxic in large doses or when taken

ingested. Do not use if pregnant.

Neroli

Neroli is another personal favorite of mine. While it's distilled from orange blossoms, don't be fooled into thinking this oil has a strictly citrus smell to it. It also smells floral and lingers around, tantalizing the nostrils. This popular oil is used mainly for its smell, but also has a number of therapeutic benefits that come along for the ride. It's relaxing and rejuvenating and is able to rebuild and repair damaged skin. Seek out unadulterated oil or you risk getting something that's only a semblance of the real thing.

Neroli Oil Information

Price:	$$ - $$$
Scent:	Lingering citrus floral.
Note:	Top to base, depending on blend.
Color:	Brown.
Source:	Orange blossoms.
Properties:	Antibacterial, anti-inflammatory, antiseptic, antispasmodic, aphrodisiac, sedative, tonic.
Good for:	Circulation, cold and flu, insomnia, scars and stretch marks, skin care, stress, wrinkles.
Contains:	Farnesol, geraniol, limonene, linalool, linalyl acetate, pinene and more.
Strength:	Mild.
Blends well with:	Lavender, lemon, spice oils.
Safety concerns:	None that I'm aware of.

Orange, Sweet

Sweet orange oil is an inexpensive oil that can be used as a deodorant and is known for its relaxing, detoxifying and warming qualities. You're going to want to buy this oil fairly early on in your journey.

Sweet Orange Oil Information

Price:	$ - $$
Scent:	Sweet citrus.
Note:	Top
Color:	Green.
Source:	Orange peels.
Properties:	Antidepressant, anti-inflammatory, antiseptic, antispasmodic, deodorant, sedative, tonic.
Good for:	Cold and flu, detox, happiness, relaxation, water retention, warmth.
Contains:	Aldehydes, limonene, linalool, myrcene, pinene and more.
Strength:	Mild, but may cause dermatitis. Dilute before use.
Blends well with:	Clary sage, citrus oils, lavender, myrrh, sandalwood.
Safety concerns:	Phototoxic. Stay away from this oil if pregnant.

Patchouli

If I had to pick a favorite oil based on scent alone, patchouli would win without a doubt. It takes a while to acclimate yourself to its scent, but the second or third time you use it, you'll find it starting to grow on you. By the 5th or 6th time, you'll find yourself looking for a reason to add it to your blends. In addition to its great smell, it has a large number of therapeutic qualities and is relatively inexpensive.

Patchouli Essential Oil

Price:	$ - $$
Scent:	Spicy and heavy.
Note:	Strong base.
Color:	Brown.
Source:	Patchouli plant.
Properties:	Antibacterial, anti-inflammatory, antimicrobial, antiseptic, antiviral, decongestant, deodorant, stimulant, tonic.
Good for:	Aches and pains, cuts and burns, dandruff, dry skin, infections, insect repellent, insect bites, oily skin, stress relief, wrinkles.
Contains:	Esters, patchoulol and more.
Strength:	Mild.
Blends well with:	Most essential oils.
Safety concerns:	Prolonged exposure to scent may cause loss of appetite. It's up to you to

decide whether this is a benefit or is detrimental.

Pine

Have you ever walked through the forest and wished you could take that fresh smell home with you? Well, you can with pine essential oil. Distilled from the needles of the pine tree, this oil has a powerful pine scent that's both invigorating and cleansing. While there are people who dilute it and apply it topically, your best bet is to diffuse it because it's strong enough to cause sensitization issues in some people.

Pine Oil Information

Price:	$
Scent:	Fresh pine.
Note:	Strong middle.
Color:	Clear.
Source:	Pine needles.
Properties:	Analgesic, antibacterial, antifungal, anti-inflammatory, antimicrobial, antiseptic, antiviral, decongestant, disinfectant, expectorant, insect repellent, stimulant.
Good for:	Aches and pains, cold and flu, fatigue, fever, insect repellent, invigorating, stress relief.
Contains:	Borneol, pinene and more.
Strength:	Strong. Best if diffused in small amounts. If you do decide to apply it topically, dilute heavily.
Blends well with:	Lavender, neroli, wood oils.

Safety concerns: Can cause sensitization issues. Avoid
                     if pregnant.

Ravensara

Ravensara essential oil comes from a plant native to Madagascar that's known to the natives as the "good leaf" tree. It has a sweet smell that some say is similar to Aniseed oil. Ravensara oil hasn't been as extensively studied or documented as many of the other essential oils, but it's traditionally been used as a general tonic thought to ward off infections and to relieve stress.

Ravensara Oil Information

Price:	$
Scent:	Similar to eucalyptus, but lighter.
Note:	Top to middle.
Color:	Yellow.
Source:	Ravensara plant.
Properties:	Analgesic, antibacterial, antiseptic, antiviral, expectorant, soothing, stimulant, tonic.
Good for:	Aches and pains, aphrodisiac, arthritis, fatigue, respiratory conditions, stress relief.
Contains:	Cineol, eucalyptol and more.
Strength:	Medium. Dilute heavily before use.
Blends well with:	Bay laurel, black pepper, citrus oils, frankincense, lavender, wood oils.
Safety concerns:	Can cause dermal irritation. Avoid use if pregnant.

Rose Otto Oil

Rose Otto oil is one of the most expensive essential oils you're going to find. The reason for the extra cost is that it takes upwards of 10,000 pounds of roses to create just a single pound of this prized oil. Don't be fooled by companies selling rose absolute oil or rose oil blends. They cost less, but pale in comparison to the fragrance of true rose otto oil.

Rose Oil Information

Price:	$$$$
Scent:	Exquisite floral.
Note:	Middle.
Color:	Yellow.
Source:	Roses.
Properties:	Analgesic, antibacterial, antifungal, antimicrobial, antiseptic, antiviral, aphrodisiac, astringent, deodorant, disinfectant, sedative, tonic.
Good for:	Cuts and burns, coughs, dry and damaged skin, emotional balancing, focus, headaches, memory, nausea, skin care, stress relief, wrinkles.
Contains:	Citronellol, geraniol, rose oxide and more.
Strength:	Mild.
Blends well with:	Most essential oils.
Safety concerns:	Do not use if pregnant.

Rosemary

Rosemary essential oil is a powerful stimulant that can be used to clear your mind and is thought to improve memory. It can also be used to help relieve congestion.

Rosemary Oil Information

Price:	$
Scent:	Medicinal and refreshing.
Note:	Middle.
Color:	Clear
Source:	Rosemary herb.
Properties:	Analgesic, antibacterial, antioxidant, antiseptic, antispasmodic, aphrodisiac, astringent, decongestant, disinfectant, expectorant, insect repellent, sedative, tonic.
Good for:	Aches and pains, cold and flu, dandruff, fatigue, focus, fluid retention, hair care, headaches, insect repellent, memory, respiratory conditions, stress relief.
Contains:	Borneol, cineole, linalol, pinene and more.
Strength:	Medium. Dilute heavily before use.
Blends well with:	Eucalyptus, lavender, peppermint, spice oils.
Safety concerns:	Do not use if pregnant or epileptic.

Sandalwood

Sandalwood essential oil is an expensive and highly sought-after oil that's sourced from the hardwood of Sandalwood trees. It has a number of therapeutic qualities and has an interesting balsamic fragrance. If you buy Sandalwood oil, make sure you get it from somewhere that practices sustainable harvesting of the hardwood used to make the oil or you may be contributing to the extinction of the species.

Sandalwood Oil Information

Price:	$$$$
Scent:	Woody and intricate.
Note:	Base.
Color:	Clear yellow.
Source:	Sandalwood hardwood.
Properties:	Antibacterial, antifungal, antiseptic, antispasmodic, aphrodisiac, astringent, decongestant, expectorant, insect repellent, sedative, tonic.
Good for:	Cold and flu, dry and damaged skin, respiratory conditions, stress relief.
Contains:	Santelenes, santolols and more.
Strength:	Mild.
Blends well with:	Jasmine, patchouli, Vetiver, wood oils.
Safety concerns:	None that I'm aware of.

Vetiver

Vetiver essential oil has a strong base note fragrance that's relaxing and soothes frayed nerves. Use it in small amounts, as it can quickly overpower a blend if you use too much. A few drops of Vetiver oil will go a long way in a blend designed to help you unwind after a long, hard day.

Vetiver Oil Information

Price:	$$
Scent:	Deep and smoky.
Note:	Base.
Color:	Brown.
Source:	Vetiver.
Properties:	Analgesic, antibacterial, antifungal, anti-inflammatory, antimicrobial, antioxidant, antiseptic, antispasmodic, sedative, tonic.
Good for:	Aches and pains, cold and flu, fatigue, headaches, insect repellent, memory, PMS, skin care, stress relief.
Contains:	Vetiverol, vetivene, vetivone and more.
Strength:	Mild, but needs to be diluted heavily because of its strong scent.
Blends well with:	Lavender, ylang ylang.
Safety concerns:	None that I'm aware of.

Therapeutic Benefits of Essential Oils

Let me begin this section by stating that essential oils should never be used to treat medical conditions without the express consent of a medical professional. You need to discuss your plans with your doctor or physician before attempting to use essential oils to ease the effect of any medical or mental condition. There may be concerns that you aren't aware of like potential side effects and negative interactions with medications you're currently taking.

The information in this section is for informational purposes and should not be used to diagnose or treat any medical condition. I can't stress enough the importance of getting the approval of your doctor prior to using essential oils and aromatherapy for therapeutic purposes. That said, I'm of the opinion that essential oils can play a role in the lives of most people and can be a tool used to ease the effects of some illnesses and health conditions. Let's take a closer look at some of the conditions that essential oils may be able to effectively help with.

NOTE: In order to make it easy for you to scale your recipe, "parts" are the unit of measure used in these recipes. To create a recipe using parts, simply replace the word "parts" with the unit of measure you want to use. If you're whipping up a small batch of an oil blend and decide to use drops as your unit of measure 5 "parts" would translate directly into 5 drops. Make sure you dilute your blends before applying them topically. Dilute to at least 5%

dilution for blends that use mild oils. For blends with oils that are possible dermal irritants, dilute to 1% or less. Always test your oil blends in a small area prior to application.

Abdominal Cramping or Pain

There are a number of reasons you may experience abdominal pain. PMS, digestive problems and the flu can all result in pain in the general area of the abdomen. Essential oils can sometimes be used to relieve this sort of pain. If the pain persists or worsens, seek immediate medical attention. You may be suffering from appendicitis or some other serious medical condition that needs to be addressed immediately.

The following blends need to be diluted with carrier oil and applied to the affected area:

Blend #1

4 parts chamomile

3 parts peppermint

Blend #2

3 parts clary sage

5 parts lavender

3 parts chamomile

Blend #3

3 parts clary sage

3 parts geranium

3 parts lavender

Blend #4

2 parts chamomile

3 parts frankincense

2 parts ginger

5 parts lavender

Acid Reflux

Some people claim to have effectively used essential oils to get rid of acid reflux issues. If you're having issues with acid reflux, the first thing you should try is upping your water intake to 8 to 10 8-ounce glasses a day. The extra water can help knock down acid reflux by diluting the acids in your stomach.

If that doesn't help, try the diluting the following oil blends to less than 2% in carrier oil and applying them to your chest:

Blend #1

3 parts chamomile

3 parts lemon

2 parts frankincense

Blend #2

3 parts chamomile

2 parts peppermint

1 part sandalwood

NOTE: Some people find that peppermint helps acid reflux, while other people claim it made their acid reflux worse. Your mileage may vary.

Blend #3

4 parts frankincense

Acne

Acne forms when the pores of the skin or the hair follicles get clogged up with dirt or other contaminants. This leads to whiteheads and blackheads, which in turn can get infected and fill with pus. There are a number of skin conditions and factors that can contribute to acne, some of which may be able to be remedied through use of essential oils.

Try diluting the following oil blends to less than 2% and applying them topically:

Blend #1

4 parts geranium

Blend #2

3 parts geranium

2 parts lemongrass

Blend #3

3 parts lavender

2 parts Cedarwood

2 parts tea tree

Addictions

Addictions are psychological attachments to a particular action or substance. There is anecdotal evidence that indicates essential oils can help ease the cravings associated with addiction. While you're probably not going to be able to quit smoking or using drugs cold turkey with no cravings just because you used essential oils, you might be able to take the edge off your cravings and make them tolerable enough to help you quit.

The following oil blends can be diluted to less than 2% and applied topically or diffused into a room to help with cravings:

Blend #1

1 part bergamot

2 parts chamomile

2 parts ylang ylang

Blend #2

3 parts grapefruit

3 parts Roman chamomile

Blend #3

3 parts lavender

2 parts sandalwood

3 parts ylang ylang

Blend #4

3 parts bergamot

3 parts clary sage

2 parts Vetiver

Blend #5

2 parts aniseed

2 parts bergamot

2 parts frankincense

Allergies

Allergy season used to be the bane of my existence. From spring through late summer, I spent my entire day sniffling, sneezing and rubbing my eyes. I'd be lying to you if I told you essential oils have completely solved my allergy woes, but they've at least made them tolerable. Essential oils don't eliminate your allergic reactions inasmuch as they ease the effects of the reactions when they do happen.

The following blends can be diffused to help ease the effects of allergic reactions:

Blend #1

2 parts lavender

3 parts lemon

2 parts peppermint

Blend #2

2 parts basil

3 parts lavender

2 parts Melissa

Blend #3

2 parts eucalyptus

1 part peppermint

2 parts tea tree

Anxiety

Constant worrying impacts your health in a number of ways. Headaches, stomachaches, ulcers and high blood pressure can all come about as a result of being overanxious for long periods of time. Essential oils with calmative and sedative properties work well to treat anxiety.

Try diluting 5 parts of lavender oil in carrier oil and applying it topically when you start to feel an attack coming on. You can also diffuse the following blends:

Blend #1

2 parts frankincense

2 parts lavender

1 part peppermint

Blend #2

2 parts cinnamon bark

2 parts Neroli

Blend #3

2 parts Sandalwood

2 parts rose

Arthritis

Arthritis is caused by inflammation of the joints that connect bones together. Essential oils that have anti-inflammatory properties can be applied topically to provide relief from this pain. The following blends can be diluted and used topically by those who suffer from arthritis pain:

Blend #1

2 parts fennel seed

2 part lemon

2 parts myrrh

Blend #2

2 parts frankincense

2 parts myrrh

3 parts peppermint

Blend #3

2 parts peppermint

3 parts lemongrass

1 part eucalyptus

Blend #4

2 parts Cedarwood

3 parts eucalyptus

2 parts Roman chamomile

Blend #5

3 parts geranium

2 parts lemongrass

Bed Bugs

The mere thought of tiny little insects sneaking out at night and sucking my blood gives me chills up and down my spine. If you're having problems with bed bugs, I really feel for you. The good news is you may be able to at least partially solve your problem through use of essential oils. Put half a cup of water into a spray bottle and add the following blend of oils to it:

10 parts lemongrass

10 parts clove

10 parts peppermint

Spray the affected areas twice a day, once in the morning and once in the afternoon. The smell is going to be rather strong, so make sure you spray a couple hours before you go to bed if you're still sleeping in the bed bug-ridden bed. Add the same mixture to your washing machine and wash all of your bedding. Spray the affected areas twice a day for up to a week.

Another oil blend you can try is:

10 parts rosemary

15 parts eucalyptus

This is also going to strong. You aren't going to want to be in the same room with this scent for at least a couple hours.

Blisters and Burns

Be it from prolonged rubbing of the skin or a burn that causes the skin to bubble up, blisters are a common occurrence. The biggest concern with blisters is they can get infected when they pop. You can help your body fight off infection by diluting and applying one of the following oil blends to your blister(s) once a day. If you have bad or extensive burning, seek medical care immediately. These blends are for minor blisters and burns only.

Blend #1

2 parts geranium

6 parts lavender

Blend #2

6 parts lavender

4 parts myrrh

Blend #3

10 parts lavender

Body Odor

Nobody wants to be the person who stinks. Essential oils can help prevent body odor by taking the battle right to the source. It seeks to eliminate the toxins and bacteria that cause the odor, while leaving you smelling fresh and clean. The following blends can be diluted and used for deodorant purposes:

Blend #1

3 parts rosemary

2 parts tea tree

Blend #2

2 parts grapefruit

3 parts lavender

2 parts tea tree

Blend #3 (For Men)

3 parts Sandalwood

2 parts tea tree

2 parts eucalyptus

Breastfeeding

You have to be extremely careful when using essential oils while breastfeeding because some oils can be passed into breast milk. Some of the stronger oils can cause digestive problems, irritability and all sorts of other problems if they're passed on in large enough amounts. Always consult with your doctor before using essential oils while breastfeeding.

Breast milk production can be a problem for some mothers. Nursing mothers may be able to increase their supply of breast milk by diluting one of the following blends and applying them topically to their breasts:

Blend #1

5 parts clary sage

5 parts geranium

Blend #2

2 parts basil

2 parts geranium

NOTE: Do not use Holy Basil for blend #2. It can actually decrease breast milk production.

Bruises

Bruising occurs when the blood vessels near the surface of the skin are broken and the bleeding can be seen just below the surface. Bruises may or may not be accompanied by pain. Essential oils can be used to help minor bruises fade away faster and to relieve the pain.

Right after a bruise starts to form, you want to dilute and apply the following blend to slow down the bleeding:

5 parts lavender

3 parts Cypress

The next day you can jumpstart the healing process by applying this blend, which is designed to improve circulation to the damaged area:

3 parts Cypress

4 parts helichrysum

3 parts geranium

If you're experiencing a lot of pain or the bruising is severe, you may have an injury that needs medical care. Seek the advice of a medical professional.

Cancer

Studies are currently underway to examine the effectiveness of various essential oils in stopping cancer dead in its tracks. What's come forth so far looks promising, but testing is still in its infancy. If you have cancer, discuss possible treatments with your doctor and an aromatherapy professional. I wouldn't be willing to bet my life on essential oils just yet, but that may change down the road.

Because treatment of cancer via essential oils is a life or death-type treatment and the stakes are so high, I can't in good conscience recommend oil blends for this sort of treatment. That said, if I were to fall victim to cancer and was told it's terminal, I would definitely look at all possible courses of treatment.

Cold and Flu

Colds and flus are lumped together into one group because the essential oil blends used to treat them are generally the same. The only difference would be adding an oil or two that combats nausea if you have a stomach flu that's causing vomiting. What I've found when using essential oils for colds and the flu is that they aren't an immediate cure like some would have you believe. Essential oils seem to dull the symptoms and make them less tolerable and recovery time may improve.

Disperse the following oil blends into a warm bath or dilute them and apply them topically:

Blend #1

2 parts eucalyptus

3 parts lavender

2 parts tea tree

Blend #2

2 parts cajeput

1 part eucalyptus

1 part pine

Blend #3

2 parts Roman chamomile

1 part lemon

2 parts tea tree

Dandruff

Dandruff occurs when your skin overproduces skin cells and oils—and then it starts to dry up and flake away. It isn't a life of death type thing, but it can feel that way when you go out in a black shirt and end up looking like someone threw a powdered doughnut at you. Dilute one of these oil blends with carrier oil and massage it into your scalp after showering:

Blend #1

3 parts lavender

3 parts lemon

2 parts rosemary

Blend #2

2 parts peppermint

3 parts rosemary

2 parts sandalwood

Depression and Sadness

The sad truth about depression is modern medicine fails to treat a vast majority of sufferers. It's difficult for doctors to prescribe medications to treat depression when they don't fully understand the science behind why people get depressed. While I would never advocate stopping medication in order to start using essential oils, those who are depressed might want to at least discuss the idea of trying essential oils with their doctors.

Depression can lead to thoughts of self-harm and suicide. If you or a loved one are severely depressed and showing signs of distress, seek help immediately. If your feelings of sadness don't go away or get worse, seek help immediately.

The following mood-balancing oil blends might help you feel a little better when you're feeling down in the dumps:

Blend #1

3 parts bergamot

3 parts lavender

3 parts Melissa

Blend #2

4 parts frankincense

3 parts Roman chamomile

2 parts Sandalwood

Blend #3

3 parts Neroli

2 parts clary sage

3 parts German chamomile

Blend #4

2 parts Neroli

2 parts rose Otto

1 part ylang ylang

Dry Skin

Dry skin can lead to chapping and cracking as it dries out past the point of no return. If you have dry, irritated skin, you want to avoid essential oils that are strongly astringent because they can dry your skin out even more. Treating dry skin with essential oils takes a two-pronged approach. Choose an essential oil blend from the list below and combine it with a carrier oil that moisturizes the skin. Massage the oil into the affected area.

Blend #1

2 parts Cedarwood

2 parts jasmine

2 parts rose otto

Blend #2

3 parts Roman chamomile

3 parts Sandalwood

Blend #3

2 parts clary sage

2 parts lavender

2 parts Sandalwood

Fatigue

Are you always tired? Do you find yourself winding down halfway through the day? Essential oils can help you feel more energetic and give you the strength you need to make it through the day. Diffuse one of the following oil blends in the morning and then periodically throughout the day when you need an energy boost.

Blend #1

2 parts rosemary

2 parts peppermint

Blend #2

2 parts bergamot

1 part eucalyptus

2 parts frankincense

Blend #3

3 parts lavender

1 part lemon

3 parts rosemary

Fever

A fever is a sign there's something wrong inside your body. When the human body experiences an infection, it raises its core temperature in an attempt to kill off the source of the infection. You can sometimes use essential oils to ward off minor infections and get rid of fevers. If you have a fever greater than 102F or if it persists for more than a day or two, you should seek medical attention.

The following oil blends can be diluted and applied topically when you have a fever:

Blend #1

2 parts peppermint

1 part rosemary

Blend #2

2 parts eucalyptus

1 part lemon

2 parts peppermint

Hair Care

Using essential oils for hair care doesn't technically fall under the scope of aromatherapy, but it bears mention. You can use essential oils in place of many of the harsh chemicals you normally put in your hair. If your hair is dry and needs moisturizing, use a carrier oil that has moisturizing benefits. If it's oily, you're going to want to use essential oils with astringent properties.

The following essential oils can be diluted and applied to your hair to keep both your hair and your scalp in good shape:

- Basil.
- Clary sage.
- Geranium.
- Lavender.
- Most citrus oils.
- Peppermint.
- Roman chamomile.
- Rosemary.
- Sandalwood.

Mix and match oils to get the benefits you need.

Headaches

Let's face it; headaches suck. If you suffer from chronic headaches or migraines, you know exactly what I mean. If aspirin or Tylenol work for you, more power to you. I'm one of those people on which they have a negligible effect. Essential oils seem to help a bit, especially for the really bad headaches.

Diffuse the following blends when you have a headache.

Blend #1

2 parts basil

3 parts frankincense

3 parts lavender

2 parts Roman chamomile

Blend #2

2 parts bergamot

4 parts lavender

1 part peppermint

Blend #3

2 parts Roman chamomile

3 parts clary sage

Hormonal Transitions (Menopause and PMS)

Essential oils are used by a number of women to help with the hormonal changes associated with both menopause and PMS.

The transition from a woman's child-bearing years into menopause can be a difficult time. In addition to the emotional burden, hot flashes and all sorts of other medical conditions can pop up as the body rebalances its hormonal levels. Essential oils can sometimes be used to help the body manage the rebalancing more efficiently and without as many problems. They can also be used to help alleviate some of the symptoms that occur.

The transition into menopause is a largely personal experience that differs greatly in both effect and emotional balance from woman to woman. There is no single blend or treatment that works for the majority of all women. Discuss essential oils with both your doctor and an aromatherapy professional to see what the best course of action for your current emotional and physical condition would be.

The same thing goes for PMS, but on a much lesser scale. Again, discuss your options with an aromatherapy practitioner to develop an effective blend for your symptoms.

Inflammation

Controlling inflammation is the key to controlling all sorts of aches, pains and ailments your body may be experiencing. Dilute the following oil blends and apply them topically to help eliminate inflammation:

Blend #1

2 parts clary sage

2 parts German chamomile

1 part fennel

Blend #2

2 parts eucalyptus

3 parts lemon

2 parts Roman chamomile

Blend #3

3 parts frankincense

2 parts myrrh

Insect Bites and Stings

Bites and stings from insects can run the gamut from extremely serious to minor irritants. If you have an infected bite or are experiencing an allergic reaction, seek immediate medical attention. If you're experiencing minor itching, burning or pain, you may be able to take care of it with essential oils. If you're attempting to treat a sting, be sure to remove the stinger prior to applying essential oil.

The following blends can be used to alleviate the itching and pain associated with insect stings and bites. Dilute it with carrier oil and apply it topically:

Blend #1

2 parts basil

3 parts lavender

2 parts peppermint

Blend #2

2 parts basil

2 parts clove

3 parts lavender

Blend #3

3 parts lemongrass

2 parts peppermint

1 part oregano

Blend #4

3 parts citronella

1 part lemongrass

2 parts peppermint

Blend #5

2 parts basil

3 parts lavender

2 parts eucalyptus

2 parts tea tree

Insect Repellant

Essential oils can be used to good effect to get rid of pesky insects, both outdoors and indoors. You can add the oils to candles, so that they repel bugs as the candle wax melts, or you can make a spray by adding the oil blend to half a cup of water and spraying it around the area you want to be bug-free. These oil blends tend to be rather hot and it's best not to apply them topically.

The following essential oil blends can be used to repel insects:

Blend #1

3 parts citronella

2 parts peppermint

Blend #2

3 parts cinnamon

1 part citronella

2 parts peppermint

Blend #3

1 part basil

2 parts eucalyptus

2 parts lemongrass

Insomnia

People with insomnia are unable to fall asleep at night or they fall asleep, but soon wake up. Those with chronic insomnia feel tired during the day and have trouble functioning normally. Essential oils can be used to help your body wind down at the end of the day. I've found these oil blends work best when added to a warm tub about an hour before bedtime. They can also be diluted and applied topically.

<u>Blend #1</u>

5 parts lavender

2 parts clary sage

<u>Blend #2</u>

4 parts frankincense

2 parts orange

3 parts ylang ylang

<u>Blend #3</u>

5 parts lavender

4 parts lemon

2 parts Sandalwood

Memory

Quick, what did you have for dinner three nights ago? If you're anything like the average person, you had trouble recalling the answer to that question. Having a bad memory can be detrimental to your life, both at home and on the job. While essential oils probably aren't going to help you memorize Pi to hundredth digit, they might help you remember the name of that important client you just met.

The following oil blends are thought to help with memory:

Blend #1

2 parts bergamot

1 part frankincense

2 parts myrrh

Blend #2

3 parts frankincense

2 parts lime

2 parts Sandalwood

1 part ylang ylang

Blend #3

2 parts clary sage

2 parts geranium

3 parts lavender

Blend #4

2 parts basil

3 parts lemon

2 parts rosemary

Oily Skin

Oily skin can lead to acne and other problems as the pores in the skin produce excess amounts of oil. Treat oily skin with astringent oils that get rid of excess oil. Dilute the following oil blends with carrier oil and apply topically:

Blend #1

2 parts lemon

2 parts peppermint

2 parts ylang ylang

Blend #2

3 parts frankincense

2 parts lime

1 part grapefruit

Blend #3

1 part lemongrass

2 parts Melissa

2 parts Neroli

Pain Relief

Aches and pains can really affect your quality of life. Sure, pain is the body's way of telling us something isn't right, but does it really have to tell us all day? I'd be more than happy only aching or hurting an hour or two a day some days. Analgesic oils shut down the receptors that send pain signals to the brain. They can be a Godsend on those days where you're really hurting. Warming oils also do a good job of alleviating pain.

The following oil blends need to be diluted heavily and applied topically for best results. Be aware that some of these oils can cause irritation. Test them in an inconspicuous area before application.

Blend #1

3 parts eucalyptus

2 parts peppermint

Blend #2

2 parts helichrysum

2 parts peppermint

Blend #3

2 parts basil

3 parts grapefruit

2 parts lavender

2 parts peppermint

Respiratory Conditions

Essential oils can be used to ease the effects of respiratory conditions like coughs, colds and bronchitis. While essential oils can provide effective relief from some respiratory conditions, they should never be used in lieu of proper medical care. Seek the advice of a medical professional prior to using essential oils to treat any major medical concern.

The following blends can be diffused for coughs:

Blend #1

2 parts eucalyptus

3 parts lemon

2 parts peppermint

Blend #2

3 parts lavender

2 parts lemon

3 parts peppermint

Blend #3

NOTE: This blend works best when inhaled as part of a steam treatment.

5 parts eucalyptus

2 parts lavender

Blend #4

3 parts eucalyptus

2 parts pine

Scar and Stretch Mark Reduction

Scars and stretch marks can really affect your quality of life. Having scars or stretch marks in visible areas can really do a number on your confidence. There are essential oil blends that may be able to help slowly but surely fade scars and stretch marks from sight.

If you have scars or stretch marks you want to get rid of, try the diluting and applying the following essential oil blends topically:

Blend #1

3 parts eucalyptus

2 parts frankincense

3 parts lavender

Blend #2

2 parts eucalyptus

3 parts geranium

Blend #3

2 parts myrrh

3 parts rose

2 parts Sandalwood

Blend #4

3 drops frankincense

2 drops geranium

3 drops jasmine

Stress Relief

The human body reacts to stressful situations by producing chemicals that place the body in fight-or-flight mode. Adrenaline and other chemicals are released that up your sense of awareness and heighten your other senses so you're prepared to deal with the situation at hand. This isn't a problem when it only takes place occasionally when the situation warrants it. It becomes a problem when a person is always stressed out because the body has difficulty adjusting to being on constant alert. It eventually begins to wear down and all sorts of problems can occur.

The following blends can be diffused, added to a bath or diluted and massaged in to help relieve stress:

Blend #1

3 parts lavender

2 parts Roman chamomile

2 parts ylang ylang

Blend #2

2 parts basil

1 part clary sage

1 part peppermint

Blend #3

3 parts lavender

2 parts Vetiver

Blend #4

3 parts bergamot

2 parts lavender

2 parts ylang ylang

Wrinkles

Ah, if only there were a fountain of youth into which we could dip whenever we notice wrinkles starting to form. A lot of the angst involved with aging would simply fade away. Essential oils aren't going to completely eliminate wrinkles and age marks, but they can help fade them out a little. Try one of the following oil blends to see if it helps:

Blend #1

2 parts frankincense

2 parts myrrh

1 parts Sandalwood

Blend #2

3 drops lavender

2 drops patchouli

3 drops rose Otto

NOTE: While you may be tempted to try to apply these oil blends to get rid of crow's feet and wrinkles around your eyes, this practice is strongly discouraged. Never apply essential oils in an area where they are in danger of coming in contact with your eyes.

Making Your Own Oil Blends

The blends listed in the previous chapter are just the tip of the iceberg when it comes to blending oils. Once you've tried a few of them, you may find you want to start making your own oil blends. There are two basic types of blending: aromatic blending and therapeutic blending.

With therapeutic blending, you choose the oils you blend together based mainly on their health benefits. If you're trying to clear up acne and oily skin, you'd look for oils with astringent qualities that are good for oily skin and combine them into a blend. While this may net you the maximum health benefit, you might find you don't particularly care for the fragrance you get from your blend. Aromatic blends, on the other hand, are blends created solely for the purpose of pleasing the nose. They smell great and have health benefits, but those benefits tend to be all over the place and not concentrated in one area.

The best aromatic blends will have oils with fragrances that complement one another as they fade in and out. The way this is done is by blending aromas that have various notes that match up well. The note of a fragrance indicates how soon you're going to smell an individual component when the fragrance reaches your nose. Top notes are the first notes you smell and they tend to fade away quickly. Middle notes come next and are a bit stronger and longer-lasting than the top notes. When the middle notes give way, the base notes take over. These are the deeper notes that stick around and linger in your nostrils.

When you blend oils to get the best fragrances, you want a combination of top, middle and base notes that all work well together. You'll see a ton of information out there that tells you which oils blend well with other oils. I've included some oils that blend well together in the oil information in this book. These are great guidelines to follow when you're a beginner, but what's important is that you find fragrances that work well for you.

Don't be afraid to experiment. Use a few drops of oil at a time in your experiments and document how many drops you're using in your blend. You don't want to create something amazing that you aren't able to recreate because you don't remember what oils you used. You're going to want to record your experiments a drop at a time. Each time you add a drop, write it down. A couple drops of oil can make a huge difference in the way a blend smells.

When you first start off, you can use the following ratios as a basic guideline for your blends:

- 20% to 40% top notes.
- 40% to 50% middle notes.
- 10% to 20% base notes.

These are only basic guidelines and rules were made to be broken. Some oils have extremely strong fragrances that can completely overpower a blend if used in more than miniscule amounts. A few drops of these oils can make a huge difference in the fragrance of a blend. Other oils have light scents that dance in and out of a fragrance. You're going to have to add more of these oils for them to make their presence known.

Creating blends is one of the most fun aspects of essential oils. You can create your own perfumes, your own skin care products and all sorts of interesting scents and blends. The sky's the limit. Don't be afraid to experiment and enjoy your journey.

www.ingramcontent.com/pod-product-compliance
Lightning Source LLC
Chambersburg PA
CBHW070639290526
45790CB00001B/141